Pre-Hospital Paediatric Life Support

THIRD EDITION

D1586842

WITHDRAWN FROM LIBRARY

BRITISH MEDICAL ASSOCIATION

1001337

Pre-Hospital Paediatric Life Support

A Practical Approach to Emergencies

THIRD EDITION

Advanced Life Support Group

EDITED BY

Alan Charters

Hal Maxwell

Paul Reavley

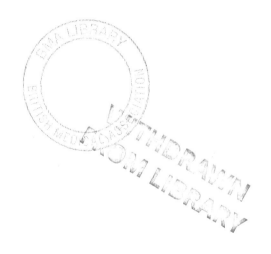

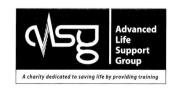

WILEY Blackwell

This edition first published 2017
© 2017 by John Wiley & Sons Ltd

Edition History
Blackwell Publishing Ltd (2e 2005)

All rights reserved. No part of this publication may be reproduced, stored in a retrieval system, or transmitted, in any form or by any means, electronic, mechanical, photocopying, recording or otherwise, except as permitted by law. Advice on how to obtain permission to reuse material from this title is available at http://www.wiley.com/go/permissions.

The right of Advanced Life Support Group (ALSG) to be identified as the author(s) of the editorial material in this work has been asserted in accordance with law.

Registered Office(s)
John Wiley & Sons, Inc., 111 River Street, Hoboken, NJ 07030, USA
John Wiley & Sons Ltd, The Atrium, Southern Gate, Chichester, West Sussex, PO19 8SQ, UK

Editorial Office
9600 Garsington Road, Oxford, OX4 2DQ, UK

For details of our global editorial offices, customer services, and more information about Wiley products visit us at www.wiley.com.

Wiley also publishes its books in a variety of electronic formats and by print-on-demand. Some content that appears in standard print versions of this book may not be available in other formats.

Limit of Liability/Disclaimer of Warranty
The contents of this work are intended to further general scientific research, understanding, and discussion only and are not intended and should not be relied upon as recommending or promoting scientific method, diagnosis, or treatment by physicians for any particular patient. In view of ongoing research, equipment modifications, changes in governmental regulations, and the constant flow of information relating to the use of medicines, equipment, and devices, the reader is urged to review and evaluate the information provided in the package insert or instructions for each medicine, equipment, or device for, among other things, any changes in the instructions or indication of usage and for added warnings and precautions. While the publisher and authors have used their best efforts in preparing this work, they make no representations or warranties with respect to the accuracy or completeness of the contents of this work and specifically disclaim all warranties, including without limitation any implied warranties of merchantability or fitness for a particular purpose. No warranty may be created or extended by sales representatives, written sales materials or promotional statements for this work. The fact that an organization, website, or product is referred to in this work as a citation and/or potential source of further information does not mean that the publisher and authors endorse the information or services the organization, website, or product may provide or recommendations it may make. This work is sold with the understanding that the publisher is not engaged in rendering professional services. The advice and strategies contained herein may not be suitable for your situation. You should consult with a specialist where appropriate. Further, readers should be aware that websites listed in this work may have changed or disappeared between when this work was written and when it is read. Neither the publisher nor authors shall be liable for any loss of profit or any other commercial damages, including but not limited to special, incidental, consequential, or other damages.

A catalogue record for this book is available from the Library of Congress and the British Library.

ISBN 9781118339763

Cover design: Wiley
Cover images: (Main image) © Jose Luis Pelaez Inc/Gettyimages; (Left inset image) © Baloncici/Gettyimages; (Middle inset image) Courtesy of the Great Western Air Ambulance Charity; (Right inset image) © artolympic/Gettyimages

Set in 10/12pt Myriad Light by SPi Global, Pondicherry, India
Printed and bound in Singapore by Markono Print Media Pte Ltd

10 9 8 7 6 5 4 3 2 1

Contents

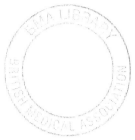

Working group

Alan Charters   RGN, RSCN, RNT, D Health Sci, MA Ed, BSc (Hons), PgDip Ed
Lead Consultant for Paediatric Emergency Care, *Portsmouth*

Sandrine Dénéréaz   Paramedic, Emergency School Director, *Lausanne, Switzerland*

Tony Little   BSc
Senior Resuscitation Practitioner/Critical Care Paramedic, *London*

Fiona Mair   MBChB, MRCGP (Assoc), DIMC (RCSEd), MRCEM (Assoc)
Emergency Medicine Associate Specialist, *Aberdeen*; member BASICS Scotland

Jeremy Mauger   MStJ, BSc(Hons), MBBS, FRCA, FFICM
Consultant in Anaesthetics and Intensive Care, *Bury St Edmunds*; HEMS Consultant, East Anglian Air
Ambulance

Hal Maxwell   BMSc (Hons), MBChB, DRCOG, FRCGP, DIMC (RCSEd)
Locum GP, Rural Dispensing Practice; member BASICS Scotland

Michael Page   BSc (Hons), Dip Sp Prac, DIMC (RCSEd), CertEd
Operational Lead (Adult) Resuscitation Services, University Hospitals Bristol NHS Foundation Trust,
Bristol; Critical Care Paramedic, South Western Ambulance Service NHS Foundation Trust

Paul Reavley   MBChB, FRCEM, FRCS(A&E)Ed, MRCGP, Dip Med Tox, RAMC
Consultant in Military Emergency and Pre-Hospital Care; Paediatric Emergency Medicine Consultant,
Bristol Royal Hospital for Children, *Bristol*

Julian M. Sandell   MBBS, MRCPI, FRCPCH, FRCEM
Consultant in Paediatric Emergency Medicine, Poole Hospital NHS Trust, *Poole*

Ronald de Vos   MD
Anesthesiologist, University Medical Center Groningen (UMCG), *Groningen, the Netherlands*

Susan Wieteska   CEO, ALSG, *Manchester*

Mark Woolcock   Consultant Paramedic, *Cornwall*

Contributors to third edition

Jim Blackburn
MBBS, BSc, MRCEM, FRCA, FIMC (RCSEd), ST5
Anaesthesia and Prehospital Emergency Medicine, *Bristol*

Vicki Brown
MCPara, MSC, DIMC (RCSEd)
Specialist Paramedic in Critical Care, Great Western Air Ambulance

Alan Charters
RGN, RSCN, RNT, D Health Sci, MA Ed, BSc (Hons), PgDip Ed
Lead Consultant for Paediatric Emergency Care, *Portsmouth*

Phil Cowburn
BSc (Hons), MBChB, FRCS, FCEM, DIMC (RCSEd)
Consultant in Emergency Medicine, Medical Director (Acute Care) Southwest Ambulance Service NHS Foundation Trust

Tony Little
BSc
Senior Resuscitation Practitioner/Critical Care Paramedic, *London*

Fiona Mair
MBChB, MRCGP (Assoc), DIMC (RCSEd), MRCEM (Assoc)
Emergency Medicine Associate Specialist, *Aberdeen*; member BASICS Scotland

Jeremy Mauger
MStJ, BSc(Hons), MBBS, FRCA, FFICM
Consultant in Anaesthetics and Intensive Care, *Bury St Edmunds*; HEMS Consultant, East Anglian Air Ambulance

Hal Maxwell
BMSc (Hons), MBChB, DRCOG, FRCGP, DIMC (RCSEd)
Locum GP, Rural Dispensing Practice; member BASICS Scotland

Michael Page
BSc (Hons), Dip Sp Prac, DIMC (RCSEd), CertEd
Operational Lead (Adult) Resuscitation Services, University Hospitals Bristol NHS Foundation Trust, *Bristol*; Critical Care Paramedic, South Western Ambulance Service NHS Foundation Trust

Paul Reavley
MBChB, FRCEM, FRCS(A&E)Ed, MRCGP, Dip Med Tox, RAMC
Consultant in Military Emergency and Pre-Hospital Care; Paediatric Emergency Medicine Consultant, Bristol Royal Hospital for Children, *Bristol*

Julian M. Sandell
MBBS, MRCPI, FRCPCH, FRCEM
Consultant in Paediatric Emergency Medicine, Poole Hospital NHS Trust, *Poole*

Ronald de Vos
MD
Anesthesiologist, University Medical Center Groningen (UMCG), *Groningen, the Netherlands*

Matthew J. C. Thomas
MBChB, FRCA, MRCP, DICM, EDIC, DIMC (RCSEd), FFICM
Consultant in Intensive Medicine, Lead Doctor, Great Western Air Ambulance

James Tooley
MBBS, MRCP, FRCPCH, DIMC (RCSEd)
Consultant in Neonatal and Paediatric Retrieval, Clinical Development Lead, Great Western Air Ambulance, *Bristol*

Christopher J. Vallis
BSc, FRCA, FRCPCH, MFSEM, CertMedEd
Consultant Paediatric Anaesthetist (retired), Royal Victoria Infirmary, *Newcastle upon Tyne*

Susan Wieteska
CEO, ALSG, *Manchester*

Mark Woolcock
Consultant Paramedic, *Cornwall*

Contributors to first and second editions

A. Charters Emergency Nursing, *Portsmouth*

T. Hodgetts Emergency Medicine, *MOD*

F. Jewkes General Practitioner and Paediatrician, *Berwickshire*

S. Levene Child Accident Prevention Trust, *London*

P. Lubas Resuscitation Training/Paramedic, *Cardiff*

I. Maconochie Paediatric Emergency Medicine, *London*

J. Mauger Anaesthetics, *Bury St Edmonds*

H. Maxwell General Practitioner, *Ballantrae*

K. McCusker Resuscitation Training/Paramedic, *Cardiff*

J. Mooney ALSG, *Manchester*

F. Moore Emergency Medicine, Ambulance Service Medical Director, *London*

P. Oakley Anaesthetics/Trauma, *Stoke*

B. Phillips ALSG, *Manchester*

P. Reavley Emergency Medicine, *Bristol*

J. Robson Paediatric Emergency Medicine, *Liverpool*

B. Stewart Paediatric Emergency Medicine, *Liverpool*

M. Vander Ambulance Service A&E Development Manager, *London*

S. Wieteska ALSG CEO, *Manchester*

M. Woolcock Pre-Hospital Practitioner, *Truro*

M. Woollard Pre-Hospital Emergency Medicine, *Middlesbrough*

Preface to third edition

The preface to the first edition of the *Pre-Hospital Paediatric Life Support* (PHPLS) manual explained that children could be saved and morbidity prevented by early and appropriate intervention. This course continues in response to that need and the need to provide a consistent, high-quality and evidence-based approach to the care of the seriously ill or injured child.

When the first course was written it grew out of the then well-established Advance Paediatric Life Support (APLS) course. As a result some of the teaching was not always transferable to the pre-hospital practitioner and their environment. Subsequent development of the course reflects the changes in resuscitation practice and recognises the demands and limitations faced by practitioners working outside hospital.

This course is aimed at the level 5 pre-hospital practitioner. An example of change is the de-emphasis of intubation and re-emphasis on good, core airway skills. The course acknowledges the role of high capability pre-hospital teams but focuses on pragmatic care delivered by the level 5 staff.

Other changes in this course reflect the introduction of current evidence-based and consensus guidelines such as the use of tranexamic acid in haemorrhage, the principle of minimal handling and the de-emphasis on cervical collars and immobilisation. The overall aim has been to maintain the high quality of the material but also reflect the changing evidence base and practice when providing care in the challenging environment that is found in the pre-hospital arena.

As always, we have aimed to keep the material consistent with the text of the current edition of the sister APLS course and some of what we have introduced in this edition of PHPLS is now being mirrored in the latest iteration of the APLS course. All knowledge is dynamic and changes will continue at pace. The Advance Life Support Group (ALSG) and its working groups will continue to develop its teaching as required.

Many, many thanks to all those who have helped with preparation and given us ideas and feedback. Thanks in advance to those of you who will continue to do so as this will ensure we keep the course relevant to your needs.

Perhaps too much has been made of the 'difficulty' of treating children in the past. Very importantly we wish to encourage you that despite fears and anxieties, you already have the knowledge and skills to help children, they are after all still members of the human race. We hope that this manual and the PHPLS course will develop you further and supply the confidence you require to treat the child in urgent need of care.

We hope you will find it useful, enjoyable and that your patients will benefit from this.

Alan Charters, Hal Maxwell and Paul Reavley
Co-Chairs PHPLS Working Group, 2017

Preface to first edition

Pre-Hospital Paediatric Life Support: The Practical Approach was written as a sister publication to *Advanced Paediatric Life Support: The Practical Approach*. It has the same objective of improving the emergency care of children, but concentrates on the first critical minutes prior to arriving at hospital.

It has been developed to fill a void in the training of personnel who have sometimes had to deal with these children with little knowledge or experience of paediatrics. Members of the pre-hospital life support working group, all of whom have extensive experience of working with children in both the pre-hospital and the hospital environments, have developed the manual in conjunction with the Joint Colleges and Ambulance Liaison Committee (JCALC) working party on paediatrics.

This manual also forms the core text of the PHPLS course, which is designed to give both medical and paramedical staff the skills and knowledge to deal with paediatric trauma and medical emergencies. The editors feel that by training together these multidisciplinary groups will both complement each other and reduce potential barriers thus developing a seamless care approach to these events.

The course is designed to dovetail with the therapies presented in APLS, building upon established and tested interventions that we hope will ultimately provide an improvement in patient outcomes.

The layout of this book begins with background information on the aetiology of illness and disease in children, followed by the assessment and basic life support of children. Specific pre-hospital considerations are then covered followed by practical skills to apply your new-found knowledge.

Emergencies in children can generate a great deal of anxiety in the children, parents and medical personnel who have to deal with them. We hope that this book will enlighten the reader on the subject of pre-hospital paediatric emergency care and provide some support to help all involved. Read it as part of the PHPLS course or as a stand-alone publication, refer to it frequently, and hopefully it will help to achieve its aim of improving the standards of paediatric life support within the pre-hospital setting.

Fiona Jewkes, Paul Lubas and Kevin McCusker
Editorial Board, December 1998

Acknowledgements

A great many people have put a lot of hard work into the production of this book and the accompanying course. The editors would principally like to thank all of the working party and contributors for their monumental efforts in the delivery of this text.

We are greatly indebted to Kirsten Baxter and Jane Mooney for their exceptional hard work and dedication towards this publication; their encouragement and guidance throughout the process has been gratefully received.

The editors gratefully acknowledge the written information and guidance received from the Great Western Ambulance Service, in particular the quick reference drugs guides reproduced in the back of the book.

We would like to thank, in advance, all of those who attend the Pre-Hospital Paediatric Life Support Course and others using this text for their continued constructive comments regarding the future development of both the course and manual.

Contact details and further information

ALSG: www.alsg.org

For details on ALSG courses visit the website or contact:
Advanced Life Support Group
ALSG Centre for Training and Development
29–31 Ellesmere Street
Swinton, Manchester
M27 0LA
Tel: +44 (0)161 794 1999
Fax: +44 (0)161 794 9111
Email: enquiries@alsg.org

Clinicians practising in tropical and under-resourced healthcare systems are advised to read *International Maternal and Child Health Care – A Practical Manual for Hospitals Worldwide* (www.mcai.org.uk) which gives details of additional relevant illnesses not included in this text.

Updates

The material contained within this book is updated on a 5-yearly cycle. However, practice may change in the interim period. We will post any changes on the ALSG website, so we advise that you visit the website regularly to check for updates (www.alsg.org/uk/phpls). The website will provide you with a new page to download.

References

All references are available on the ALSG website www.alsg.org/uk/phpls

On-line feedback

It is important to ALSG that the contact with our providers continues after a course is completed. We now contact everyone 6 months after their course has taken place asking for on-line feedback on the course. This information is then used whenever the course is updated to ensure that the course provides optimum training to its participants.

How to use your textbook

The anytime, anywhere textbook

Wiley E-Text

Your textbook comes with free access to a **Wiley E-Text: Powered by VitalSource** version – a digital, interactive version of this textbook which you own as soon as you download it.

Your **Wiley E-Text** allows you to:

Search: Save time by finding terms and topics instantly in your book, your notes, even your whole library (once you've downloaded more textbooks)

Note and Highlight: Colour code, highlight and make digital notes right in the text so you can find them quickly and easily

Organize: Keep books, notes and class materials organized in folders inside the application

Share: Exchange notes and highlights with friends, classmates and study groups

Upgrade: Your textbook can be transferred when you need to change or upgrade computers

Link: Link directly from the page of your interactive textbook to all of the material contained on the companion website

The **Wiley E-Text** version will also allow you to copy and paste any photograph or illustration into assignments, presentations and your own notes.

To access your Wiley E-Text:

- Find the redemption code on the inside front cover of this book and carefully scratch away the top coating of the label.
- Go to **https://online.vitalsource.co.uk** and log in or create an account. Go to Redeem and enter your redemption code to add this book to your library.
- Or to download the Bookshelf application to your computer, tablet or mobile device go to **www.vitalsource.com/ software/bookshelf/downloads**.
- Open the Bookshelf application on your computer and register for an account.
- Follow the registration process and enter your redemption code to download your digital book.
- If you have purchased this title as an e-book, access to your **Wiley E-Text** is available with proof of purchase within 90 days. Visit **http://support.wiley.com** to request a redemption code via the 'Live Chat' or 'Ask A Question' tabs.

The VitalSource Bookshelf can now be used to view your Wiley E-Text on iOS, Android and Kindle Fire!

- **For iOS:** Visit the app store to download the VitalSource Bookshelf: **http://bit.ly/17ib3XS**
- **For Android and Kindle Fire:** Visit the Google Play Market to download the VitalSource Bookshelf: **http://bit.ly/BSAAGP**

You can now sign in with the email address and password you used when you created your VitalSource Bookshelf Account.

Full E-Text support for mobile devices is available at: **http://support.vitalsource.com**

We hope you enjoy using your new textbook. Good luck with your studies!

CHAPTER 1
Introduction

Learning outcomes

After reading this chapter, you will be able to:
- Describe the focus of the PHPLS course
- Identify the important differences in children and the impact of these on the management of emergencies

---

Over the last two decades there has been a substantial reduction in childhood mortality across the world. This has been related to improvements in many areas such as maternal education, access to clean water, access to food, immunisation against an increasing number of infectious conditions and improved access to healthcare services. Even conditions such as human immunodeficiency virus (HIV) infections have potentially come under control with the development of highly effective antiretroviral therapeutic regimes. However, children across the world continue to suffer potentially life-threatening acute illness (sometimes on a background of chronic illness) and injury. The Pre-Hospital Paediatric Life Support (PHPLS) course is directed at training healthcare workers to recognise life-threatening illness or injury in children; to provide effective emergency intervention; and to ensure that children are directed to the appropriate place for ongoing definitive management of the condition as soon as possible. This approach is potentially applicable in many different settings across the world.

1.1 Principles

There are a number of principles that underpin this approach. Pre-hospital healthcare professionals must:

- Be reassured that acquired experience and skills are transferable to children's illness and trauma management but be aware of the important areas of difference and your own development needs
- Adopt and rehearse a structured approach to the assessment and management of children's illness and injury
- Ensure appropriate paediatric equipment is carried and be familiar with its use
- Include paediatric training and education in professional development and clinical governance processes

Physiological differences

Most clinical medicine is taught with the underlying assumption that adults best exemplify 'normal' in health. This is perhaps justified by the reality that in most parts of the world the majority of the population is made up of adults, but in poorer countries up to 40% of the population may be made up of children (depending on how children are defined). Thus it is important to highlight where children are different to adults in terms of physiology, pathophysiology and responses to various interventions (see Section 1.2). A key area of successful paediatric care is understanding that children physiologically compensate extremely well in acute illness and injury. A consequence of this is that an inexperienced practitioner may not recognise the early stages of disease or injury, and without intervention the child may deteriorate to the point of decompensation. In children decompensation is rapid and difficult to reverse; paediatric cardiac arrest represents the end of a long and missed opportunity to intervene. Thus particular attention has to be paid to timely and effective support of the respiratory and cardiovascular systems in particular.

Pre-Hospital Paediatric Life Support: A Practical Approach to Emergencies, Third Edition. Edited by Alan Charters, Hal Maxwell and Paul Reavley.
© 2017 John Wiley & Sons Ltd. Published 2017 by John Wiley & Sons Ltd.

Children come in a range of sizes, and a consequence of this is the constant requirement to adjust all therapy, interventions and selection of equipment or consumable to the size of the particular patient (see Table 1.1).

Relationship between disease progression and outcomes

The further a disease process is allowed to progress, the worse the outcome is likely to be. The outcomes for children who have a cardiac arrest out of hospital are generally poor because cardiac arrest is rarely related to a sudden cardiac arrhythmia, but more commonly is a sequel of hypoxaemia and/or shock with associated organ damage, dysfunction and often irreversible decompensation (Figure 1.1). By the time that cardiac arrest occurs, there has already been substantial damage to end organs. This is in contrast to situations (more common in adults) where the cardiac arrest was the consequence of cardiac arrhythmia – with preceding normal perfusion and oxygenation. Thus the focus of the course is on early recognition and effective management of potentially life-threatening problems before there is progression to respiratory and/or cardiac arrest.

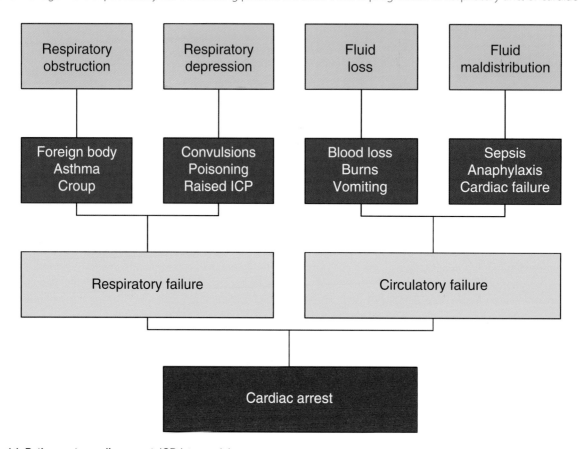

Figure 1.1 Pathways to cardiac arrest. ICP, intracranial pressure

Standardised structure for assessment and stabilisation

The use of a standardised structure for resuscitation provides benefits in many areas. Firstly it provides a structured approach to a critically ill child who may have multiple problems. The standardised approach enables the provision of a standard working environment, ensuring that all the necessary equipment is available as required. By focusing attention on life-threatening issues and dealing with these in a logical sequence it is possible to stabilise the child's condition quickly. The use of the standardised structure enables the entire team to know what is likely to be expected of them and in what sequence.

There may well be discussion around the optimum sequence of resuscitation, but in this course a particular approach has been accepted as being reasonable, and most in keeping with the available research information. It is likely that aspects of this approach will change over time, and in fact it may be appropriate to modify the approach in particular working environments and contexts.

Once basic stabilisation has been achieved, it is then appropriate to investigate the underlying diagnoses and proceed to definitive therapy. Occasionally, definitive therapy (such as surgical intervention) may be a component of the resuscitation.

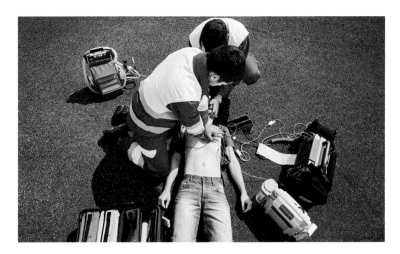

Figure 1.2 PHPLS in action

Resource management

There is increasing realisation that provision of effective emergency treatment depends on the development of teams of healthcare providers who are able to work together in a coordinated and appropriately directed way (Figure 1.2). Thus part of training in paediatric life support must focus on understanding how the human resources available for a particular resuscitation episode can be utilised most effectively.

Early transfer to appropriate teams for definitive management

It is clear that within the pre-hospital setting you are unlikely to be able to provide anything other than initial assessment and early resuscitative measures (pre-hospital critical care teams may be able to provide more than this). Definitive management will need to be provided in the most appropriate setting available. This will require decisions about where to transfer, what mode of transfer (i.e. road ambulance or helicopter) or whether to seek a retrieval team to assist. These will all depend on particular circumstances in which you find yourself.

1.2 Important differences in children

Children vary in weight, size, shape, intellectual ability and emotional response. At birth a child is, on average, a 3.5 kg, 50 cm long individual with small respiratory and cardiovascular reserves and an immature immune system. They are capable of limited movement, exhibit limited emotional responses and are dependent upon adults for all their needs. Fourteen or more years later at the other end of childhood, the adolescent may be a 50 kg, 160 cm tall person who looks physically like an adult, is often exhibiting a high degree of independent behaviour but who may still require support in ways that are different to adults.

Competent management of a seriously ill or injured child who may fall anywhere between these two extremes requires a knowledge of these anatomical, physiological and emotional differences and a strategy of how to deal with them.

Weight

The most rapid changes in weight occur during the first year of life. An average birth weight of 3.5 kg will have increased to 9.5 kg by the age of 1 year. After that time weight increases more slowly until the pubertal growth spurt.

As most drugs and fluids are given as the dose per kilogram of body weight, it is important to determine a child's weight as soon as possible. Clearly the most accurate method for achieving this is to weigh the child on scales; however, in an emergency, this may be impracticable. Very often, especially with infants, the child's parents or carer will be aware of a recent weight. If this is not possible, various formula or reference guides are available, e.g. the Joint Royal Colleges and Ambulance Liaison Committee (JRCALC) page per age handbook or the page per age resource included in the Appendix to this manual. Various formulae may also be used although they should be validated to the population in which they are being used.

Table 1.1 Normal ranges

Age	Guide weight (kg)	RR At rest Breaths per minute 5th–95th centile	HR Beats per minute 5th–95th centile	BP Systolic 5th centile	50th centile	95th centile
Birth	3.5	25–50	120–170	65–75	80–90	105
1 month	4.5					
3 months	6.5	25–45	115–160			
6 months	8	20–40	110–160			
12 months	9.5			70–75	85–95	
18 months	11	20–35	100–155			
2 years	12	20–30	100–150	70–80	85–100	110
3 years	14		90–140			
4 years	16		80–135			
5 years	18			80–90	90–110	110–120
6 years	21		80–130			
7 years	23					
8 years	25	15–25	70–120			
9 years	28					
10 years	31					
11 years	35					
12 years	43	12–24	65–115	90–105	100–120	125–140
14 years	50		60–110			
Adult	70					

BP, blood pressure; HR, heart rate; RR, respiratory rate.

If a child's age is known the normal ranges table here will provide you with an approximate weight (Table 1.1). This will allow you to then prepare the appropriate equipment and drugs for the child's arrival in hospital. Whatever the method, it is essential that the carer is sufficiently familiar with it to be able to use it quickly and accurately under pressure. When arriving at an incident, you should quickly review the child's size to check if it is much larger or smaller than predicted. If you have a child that looks particularly large or small for their age, you can go up or down one age group.

As the child's weight increases with age the size, shape and proportions of various organs also change (Figure 1.3).

Physiological differences in different sized children include the following.

Respiratory

The infant has a relatively greater metabolic rate and oxygen consumption. This is one reason for an increased respiratory rate. However, the tidal volume remains relatively constant in relation to body weight (5–7 ml/kg) through to adulthood. The work of breathing is also relatively unchanged at about 1% of the metabolic rate, although it is increased in the pre-term infant.

The infant's compliant chest wall leads to prominent sternal and subcostal recession when the airways are obstructed or lung compliance decreases. It also allows the intrathoracic pressure to be less 'negative'. This reduces small-airway patency. As a result, the lung volume at the end of expiration is similar to the closing volume (the volume at which small-airway closure starts to take place).

The combination of high metabolic rate and oxygen consumption with low lung volumes and limited respiratory reserve means that infants in particular will desaturate much more rapidly than adults. This is an important consideration during procedures such as endotracheal intubation.

The immature infant lung is also more vulnerable to insult. Following prolonged respiratory support of a pre-term infant, chronic lung disease of the newborn may cause prolonged oxygen dependence. For example, infants who have suffered from bronchiolitis can remain 'chesty' for a year or more. Table 1.1 shows respiratory rate by age at rest.

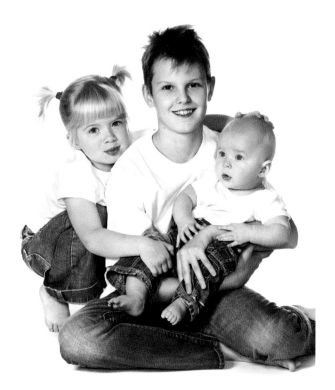

Figure 1.3 Differences in children

Cardiovascular

The infant has a relatively small stroke volume (1.5 ml/kg at birth) but has the highest cardiac index seen at any stage of life (300 ml/min/kg). Cardiac index decreases with age and is 100 ml/min/kg in adolescence and 70–80 ml/min/kg in the adult. At the same time the stroke volume increases, the heart gets bigger and the amount of muscle mass relative to connective tissue increases. As cardiac output is the product of stroke volume and heart rate, these changes underlie the heart rate changes seen during childhood in Table 1.1.

Normal systolic pressures are also shown in Table 1.1.

As the stroke volume is small and relatively fixed in infants, cardiac output is principally related to heart rate. The practical importance of this is that the response to volume therapy is blunted when normovolaemic because stroke volume cannot increase greatly to improve cardiac output. By the age of 2 years myocardial function and response to fluid are similar to those of an adult.

Systemic vascular resistance rises after birth and continues to do so until adulthood is reached. This is reflected in the changes seen in blood pressure (Table 1.1).

Immune function

At birth the immune system is immature and, consequently, infants are more susceptible than older children to many infections such as bronchiolitis, septicaemia, meningitis and urinary tract infections. Maternal antibodies acquired across the placenta provide some early protection but these progressively decline during the first 6 months. These are replaced slowly by the infant's antibodies as he or she grows older, sometimes in response to immunisation. Breastfeeding provides increased protection against respiratory and gastrointestinal infections.

Psychological

Children vary enormously in their intellectual ability and their emotional response. A knowledge of child development assists in understanding a child's behaviour and formulating an appropriate management strategy. Particular challenges exist in communicating with children and as far as possible easing their fear of the circumstances they find themselves in.

Communication

Infants and young children either have no language ability or are still developing their speech. This causes difficulty when symptoms such as pain need to be described. Even children who are usually fluent may remain silent when unwell or in pain. Information has to be gleaned from the limited verbal communication, and from the many non-verbal cues (such as facial expression and posture) that are available. Older children are more likely to understand aspects of their illness and treatment and so be reassured by adequate age-appropriate communication.

Fear

Many clinical situations engender fear in children. This causes additional distress to the child and adds to parental anxiety. Physiological parameters, such as pulse rate and respiratory rate, are often raised because of it, and this in turn makes clinical assessment of pathological processes, such as shock, more difficult.

Children can be irrational and tend to be more fearful in the presence of injury and illness. Medical examination and intervention will be scary to the majority of children. Adolescents will have different health beliefs and need careful communication to engage in healthcare. Knowledge dispels fear and it is therefore important to explain things as clearly as possible to the child. Explanations must be phrased in a way that the child can understand. Play can be used to do this in younger children (e.g. applying a bandage to a teddy first), and also helps to maintain some semblance of normality in a strange and stressful situation. Finally, parents must be allowed to stay with the child at all times (including during resuscitation if at all possible); their absence from the child's bedside will only add further fears, both to the child and to the parents themselves. Importantly, parents too must be supported and fully informed at all times.

1.3 Summary

The Pre-Hospital Paediatric Life Support course is focused on providing training for healthcare professionals in the recognition and management of life-threatening illness in children; in recognition and initial management of important underlying conditions; and appropriate referral to teams that are able to provide definitive intervention. In this process it is also essential to remember the needs of the child's family and to support the clinical team.

You should also be aware that there are some important differences in children:

- Absolute size and relative body proportions change with age
- Observations of children must be related to their age
- Therapy in children must be related to their age and weight
- The special psychological needs of children must be considered

CHAPTER 2
Scene management in incidents involving children

Learning outcomes

After reading this chapter, you will be able to:
- Describe the CSCATTT structure and approach to scene management
- Communicate using the ATMISTER format

A logical approach to scene management is essential in paediatric incidents, as it is very easy for emotions to cloud judgement when children are involved. This may endanger the responder, patient and others alike.

Most responses will be to the home environment, which is usually a simple and safe scene. In this case the pre-hospital responder will be free from distraction to establish rapport and deal with the child's healthcare needs and parental or carer's emotional needs.

Incidents outside the home in public areas are more complex for a variety of reasons, and an understanding of structured incident response is important. A simple, systematic approach to the management of any incident can be remembered as:

CSCATTT

C	Command
S	Safety
C	Communication
A	Assessment
T	Triage
T	Treatment
T	Transport

Command

Depending on the nature of the incident, scenes will often involve several other teams, including ambulance, fire and police. Each will have its own commander; therefore cooperation and coordination are important to achieve timely care and transport.

Command and control of an incident is often implicit. In some instances it may be necessary to assert authority and gain control of a group of people before being able to manage a casualty effectively. However, pre-hospital teams need a good understanding of how different agencies exert command and control. Who has primacy may vary with the task and situation. Often the police have assumed authority but this may be surrendered in the case of a specific hazard such as fire or chemicals in which case the fire service will assume control.

Safety

Safety is paramount and personal safety has priority over all else. Personal safety is increased by wearing appropriate personal protective equipment. For the medic attending a child in a stable environment, this may be no more than disposable gloves. However this must be escalated to match on-scene hazards and rescuers must have appropriate protective equipment in order not to become a casualty themselves.

Safety of a roadside scene is achieved by parking to protect the scene. Where necessary, the police will provide a scene cordon, control traffic and protect the scene for forensic investigation if required. Fire and rescue services will deal with immediate hazards such as fire, chemical and fuel leaks and entrapment.

Safety of any casualties should be subordinate to personal safety and scene safety. It is easy to imagine the situation where the temptation exists to rush in and help a vulnerable child at the expense of personal safety.

Communication

Poor communication is the principle failing of scene management. Remember you must communicate not only internally with your team but externally with other agencies at the scene and also elsewhere. Communication should be short, to the point and clear.

The receiving hospital must be alerted as soon as is practicable and all relevant information passed in a succinct, accurate and clear manner.

Teams of specialist staff may be involved in the treatment of a seriously ill or injured child and they require time to prepare personnel and resources for the arrival of the child. It is very common for receiving hospitals not to be alerted, resulting in delayed and uncoordinated treatment of the child on arrival at hospital.

Communication with the receiving hospital must be treated as an integral part of the child's treatment in the same manner as the primary or secondary assessment. The aim is to provide seamless treatment between the pre-hospital and hospital settings, resulting in the best possible provision of care to the patient. The commonly used format for pre-hospital communication is the AT MISTER.

AT MISTER	
A	Age and sex
T	Time of incident
M	Mechanism of injury
I	Injury suspected
S	Signs including vital signs and GCS score
T	Treatment so far
E	Estimated time of arrival to the emergency department
R	Requirements, e.g. bloods, specialist services, tiered response, ambulance call sign

This should be practised in training serials until it is smooth and coherent.

Assessment

Scene assessment may be straightforward if responding to one child in the home environment. However, a rapid assessment on approach is recommended to assess safety issues, the atmospherics of the situation and the mood of those around the situation. There is often a degree of heightened anxiety surrounding a sick or injured child and this can escalate to anger with clumsy handling of the situation. Assessment of the surrounding scene can be vital in situations where non-accidental injury is suspected and your observations could prove vital in the safeguarding of children.

At scenes of accidents such as road incidents, a rapid assessment of the number and severity of casualties is required. Remember, children are small and can be hard to find at a scene. The presence of a car seat, toys or a buggy may indicate the presence of a child. Children can be ejected, thrown into footwells, hidden under wreckage, etc. and it is vital that their presence is either excluded or confirmed as soon as possible. Look everywhere.

Triage

When the number or types of casualties exceed resources available, it is essential to prioritise for treatment. This is covered in detail in Chapter 13.

Treatment

Treatment at the scene is generally limited to whatever immediate life-saving intervention is required. Teams with paediatric critical care capability may decide to do more at the scene; this goes against the instinctive scoop and run approach. For example, in the case of cardiac arrest, the team's capability may be as good or even exceed the destination unit and they may chose to treat at the scene for longer than lower capability teams would. Sometimes more effective care can be provided statically, at the scene, than on the move.

Transport

Transportation of children falls within two main categories. Primary transfer involves the child being moved to the initial receiving hospital and secondary transfer is usually between the initial receiving hospital and another medical facility or specialist (paediatric) treatment centre.

It is important not to delay the patient at the scene unduly, but it is also important that a child is not transferred between locations without adequate preparation and planning. Depending on the situation and the patient's condition, this may take from minutes to hours. Unnecessarily delaying transfer and treatment may worsen the likelihood of long-term survival.

A systematic approach must be employed to assess the child's condition and whether to treat on the scene or move to hospital without delay:

Systematic approach to out of hospital patient care

- Primary assessment
- Resuscitation
- Secondary assessment
- Emergency treatment
- Definitive care

Triaging transport

Determining the most appropriate destination for ill or injured children to be safely transported to is an important consideration that can impact on prognosis. You may have local guidance or regional networks in place to follow when deciding where to transport paediatric patients.

The child, parents and carers

Most children will come with at least one parent or carer and frequently more. They will be at best anxious and at worst hysterical, that is why they have called for help. Your calmness and professionalism will support them and anything less than this will only concern them further. Where at all possible, keep the parent at the child's side, even if the child is critically ill or in cardiac arrest. This may be uncomfortable for the provider but it is crucial for the parent to be there at that time and this will comfort the patient.

Some people are naturally adept with children, others are not. Try to imagine how your 5-year-old self would respond to two adults dressed in odd and sometimes lurid uniforms, arriving in your home with bags and machines. Be nice, be gentle and remember personal dignity is secondary to the requirement to form a quick trust between you, the child and the carer. Have a strategy.

CHAPTER 3
Preparation

Learning outcomes

After reading this chapter, you will be able to:
- Consider the needs of the paediatric patient when preparing for delivery of pre-hospital care

3.1 Introduction

Dealing with children who are ill can be challenging in comfortable, well lit surroundings with a full complement of staff and equipment. Dealing with such children on your own, in the home or at the site of injury can be particularly challenging.

In hospital the main decisions in dealing with an ill child are twofold:

- What do I need to do now?
- Which colleagues do I call on for help?

When assessing the child in the pre-hospital setting, there are several more decisions including:

- What help do I need and where can I get this help?
- How do I transport the child and with what urgency?
- To which facility do I send the child?

Additionally, in the pre-hospital setting each provider brings a different level of skill and ability to the task of caring for the child. This section does not, therefore, attempt to be a step-by-step manual, but rather is presented as a series of key points. These should be personalised for your own circumstances. Prior preparation and a detailed knowledge of the following areas will prevent failure when faced with injured and unwell children.

The areas covered in this section are:

- Resources
- Equipment
- Facts, figures and formulae
- Training and governance

Pre-Hospital Paediatric Life Support: A Practical Approach to Emergencies, Third Edition. Edited by Alan Charters, Hal Maxwell and Paul Reavley.
© 2017 John Wiley & Sons Ltd. Published 2017 by John Wiley & Sons Ltd.

Resources

In considering the resources, you need to look at the following:

Personnel

Consider the skill mix in your team and identify the limitations you have. The additional capability you may need should be addressed through personal and team development. There may be other medical assets in your area of operations, such as critical care teams, and a good knowledge of their capabilities and how to access them is required.

Hospitals/medical facilities – consider what hospitals/medical assets are in your locality and what services and facilities they provide. Consider not only their medical care capabilities but also their extraction and transport capabilities. Be aware of any local, regional and supra-regional networks such as ones for burns or trauma, and how to access them. It is vital to keep a record of contact telephone numbers and call signs.

Equipment

For simplicity, consider equipment needs in terms of the <C>ABCDE approach. Ask the question, do you have appropriate paediatric-specific equipment for a range of children in each of these areas?

<C> = Catastrophic haemorrhage

Catastrophic haemorrhage equipment such as arterial tourniquets and pelvic splints can be difficult to fit to smaller children. Review the devices you carry in view of their suitability for children. Compression dressings and haemostatic dressings are not generally size specific.

A = Airway

Include in this simple airway adjuncts, supraglottic airway devices, laryngoscopes, endotracheal tubes, suction and tube holders.

B = Breathing

Include bag–valve–mask devices, pocket masks, oxygen delivery units, ventilation circuits and end tidal monitoring devices.

C = Circulation

Consider here how you will achieve vascular access and what you will give. Carry a range of paediatric cannulas and intraosseous devices. Be very familiar with intraosseous insertion sites. Do not forget appropriate dressings to protect and stabilise the access.

D = Drugs

This list will vary depending on skills, training and protocols but it is essential to carry a range of drugs in appropriate preparations for all age ranges. Remember that drugs can be given by the intravenous (IV), intraosseous (IO), intranasal (IN), intramuscular (IM), subcutaneous (SC) and per rectum (PR) routes and to carry the correct equipment to enable this. The intranasal route is very underutilised but is well proven and safe; to facilitate this route carry mucosal atomiser devices.

Facts, figures and formulae

In order to recognise the abnormal it is essential to have normal values at your fingertips, preferably accessible on a smartphone application or as prepared age/weight charts (see Appendix). When stress increases, memory decreases and errors can be made.

All calculations of drug doses, fluids, etc. start with the weight of the child in kilograms. While there is an easy formula to help calculate this, do not forget simple approaches like asking the mother. It is likely, however, that most mothers in the UK will quote the weight of young children in pounds and older children in stones. For pre-hospital care it is perfectly acceptable to use the very simple and traditional formula:

$$\text{Weight in kg} = (\text{Age} + 4) \times 2$$

To convert stones or pounds to kilos the conversions are:

$$1\,\text{kg} = 2.2\,\text{lb}$$

$$1\,\text{stone} = 6.3\,\text{kg}$$

See the Appendix for example reference tables. Many pre-hospital emergency care providers carry 'page per age' tables with all the required physiological, drug and equipment references required for a child of a specific age. There are also various pre-hospital measurement tapes available, which act as a helpful aide memoire also. Make your own choice, but have something weather proofed in your bag to aid your recall when needed.

Training and governance

In areas where we get less regular hands on practice, the only opportunity to keep skills and knowledge up to date is through individual and unit teaching and training. The less we do something for real, the more we need to practise it. Paediatric topics and skills should be included in unit training programmes. In order to direct exactly what knowledge and training is required, it is vital that all significant paediatric cases are reviewed through the governance process. This includes the hot debrief and clinical governance meetings.

CHAPTER 4

Assessment and immediate management of the seriously ill or injured child

Learning outcomes

After reading this chapter, you will be able to:
- Describe how to recognise the seriously ill or injured child
- Describe the structured approach to the assessment of the seriously ill or injured child
- Describe the structured approach to resuscitation of the seriously ill or injured child

4.1 Assessment

Introduction

Children compensate well physiologically in times of stress and, thus, the signs of serious illness may be subtle.

Assessment has two elements, namely assessment of the scene and assessment of the ill or injured child.

Scene assessment

When considering injury, assessment of the scene can give a lot of information about what to expect when it comes to assessing the child. This is less commonly considered but equally valid when dealing with an ill child.

All scene assessment starts with one's own safety, making sure that there are no immediate dangers to the healthcare practitioner seeing the child. Following this, when approaching the child it is essential to 'read the scene' for clues as to the problem. For example, in the case of a road traffic collision where a child is knocked off a bike by a car, you will look at the vehicle involved, the areas of damage to the vehicle, the damage to the bike and the relative positions of the car, bike and child to gain an idea of what part of the child's body sustained the impact, how much force the child was subject to and thus the potential injuries.

When seeing an ill child in his or her home, the same principles are followed. You will be aware of your safety as you approach, for example looking for evidence of dogs in the house. You will also observe the demeanour of the family – is mum waiting at the door when you get there looking anxious and distraught or are the family indifferent and untroubled. As part of the

Pre-Hospital Paediatric Life Support: A Practical Approach to Emergencies, Third Edition. Edited by Alan Charters, Hal Maxwell and Paul Reavley.
© 2017 John Wiley & Sons Ltd. Published 2017 by John Wiley & Sons Ltd.

scene assessment consider also the overall appearance of the house, is it clean and well ordered or chaotic and dirty. These factors will give clues to potential illness severity, to family parenting and coping skills and may hint that there are other underlying stresses in the house that impact upon the care of the child.

In summary, when approaching a child be aware of any danger to yourself first and foremost, then assess the scene for clues as to the mechanism of injury and factors influencing the care of the child.

Initial assessment of illness and injury

The initial assessment of an ill or injured child will follow the < C > ABCDE approach.

The general appearance of the child can often give a rapid and accurate assessment as to what kind of medical intervention is going to be required. Is the child happy and alert? A child who is pale in colour, lethargic or floppy in a mother's arms is more likely to need urgent medical intervention and transport than a child who is laughing and reaching out for toys. More valuable information can be learned by merely observing a child than by immediately trying to perform a detailed examination. This is particularly so in toddlers, who can be very difficult to examine because of their innate fear of strangers. The healthcare professional should try to work at the same height as the child – bending over a child may be threatening. Smiling and cheerfulness will be very reassuring, especially when using equipment such as a stethoscope. In situations that are not life threatening, bring play into the assessment. Clothes should only be removed if this is essential and only from one area at a time. The exception is when the child feels very hot, in which case minimal loose clothing is appropriate to facilitate cooling.

There are a few principles to follow when dealing with children:

1. Never lie to or surprise children. If you are going to perform a procedure, particularly something unpleasant, explain in an age-appropriate way the reason for needing to do so and tell the child that the procedure will/may hurt. Lying to or not involving a child about what is going to happen could lead to that child losing trust in all those subsequently caring for them. However, the time taken to explain something to the child needs to be balanced against the timeliness of extraction.
2. Always involve the parents in the assessment. In the majority of age groups, having the child sit on a parent's knee, or getting a parent to distract the child, will not only help to reassure the child, but will make the parents feel that they are doing something and this, in itself, will reassure both them and their child. Remember that parents often feel very helpless and may feel guilty if a child has an injury. If the situation permits, always try to keep the parents and the child together. A young child will not understand why his or her parents are being removed, and the fears they already have will be compounded by the fact that they may fear they will never see their family again.
3. Never be angry with children, however uncooperative they may become while you are attempting to help. Anger will not help to gain the child's cooperation, may distress the child further and will almost certainly also distress the parents. Calm encouragement and a kind smiling face will do a lot to reassure both the parents and the patient, however you are feeling.
4. Always involve children in discussions regarding their care, especially older children. Also remember that disabled children may comprehend more than you appreciate. It is very demeaning for a child to be totally ignored while the parents have the procedure explained to them. This attitude does not engender trust.

There are additional considerations in assessing children of different ages.

Infants

Some babies will be crying already when you approach them and others may become upset by attempts to examine them. Well children are usually consolable if upset. If a child remains calm during examination or can be settled with soothing, this is often termed 'handles well', and may be reassuring. One possible feature of serious illness is irritability or an inconsolable infant. The pitch and nature of the cry may be different or abnormal; parents are very alert to this. It is important to take parental awareness of the presence of abnormality very seriously and seek further assessment. Feeling the fontanelle (or 'soft spot') can be a helpful additional sign. It is normally soft. Tension of the fontanelle may indicate raised intracranial pressure; however, the fontanelle will also become tense when the infant is crying. A sunken fontanelle may indicate dehydration.

In infants over the age of 6 or 7 months, it may be better to conduct the examination, where possible, with the child on the parent's knee (Figure 4.1). Although this makes examination of some parts, such as the abdomen, difficult, you will get more information from examining a cooperative child in this position than from a hysterical child who has been prised away from his or her mother.

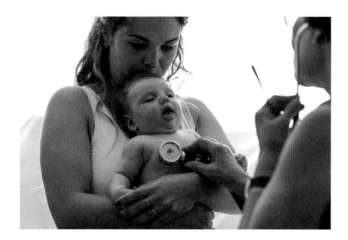

Figure 4.1 Approaching an infant for examination

Generally, it is better to examine the parts of the anatomy that require relative quiet first, in case the infant later becomes upset by the examination. This still allows assessment and examination of the airway, breathing and circulation in the conventional order of ABC. It is usually best to leave examination of painful areas or the ear, nose and throat until last.

It is not always appropriate, or necessary, to examine every infant from top to toe, exposing every inch of the body unless for a specific reason, e.g. a skin rash is being sought. Indeed, it may actually be harmful, delaying transport and allowing the child to become cold and frightened.

Toddlers

Toddlers present many of the difficulties of younger infants during examination, but in addition there are two extra points to remember.

Firstly, they tend to be increasingly wary of strangers and, secondly, some children of this age can be particularly willful and determined not to be examined. Generally, this is a sign that they are not seriously ill and this should be quite reassuring to the examiner, although it may be inconvenient. Often a gentle approach, at eye level (Figure 4.2), explaining to the child in terms he or she can understand, may be adequately reassuring to allow examination. It is particularly important to get the parent to help you to reassure and to hold the child.

Allowing a frightened child to play with instruments that will be used can often avert the fear which the child may experience. If the child does become frightened and uncooperative, it is generally best to restrict the examination to that which is absolutely essential. It may even be necessary to restrict the examination to only that of the general appearance, as described above. This is particularly important when upper airway obstruction is being considered, as in croup or suspected foreign body inhalation. Agitation may lead to complete airway obstruction and respiratory arrest in these circumstances. It is very important that no attempt is made to examine the mouth or throat if the child has stridor.

(a)

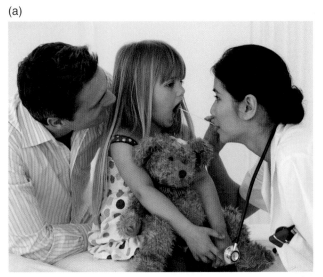

(b)

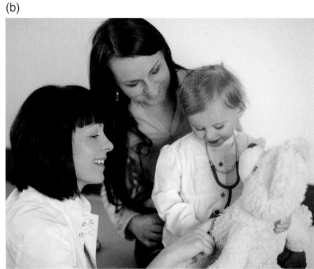

Figure 4.2 Approaching a child for examination

If the child does become agitated, it will only make matters worse if the examiner becomes impatient. To continue with kind words and smiles may do much more to alleviate the situation than showing the impatience which the examiner may be feeling.

School children

As communication is easier in this group one would expect that cooperation would be greater, and in general it is. However, children sometimes regress in times of stress and become apparently quite unreasonable. In these circumstances it is important to remain patient and calm. Always try to include the child or young person in the conversation – it is very rude to pretend they are not there! If an older child seems unduly frightened, he or she may be much happier sitting on a parent's knee (Figure 4.3).

(a)

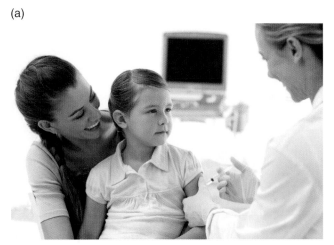

(b)

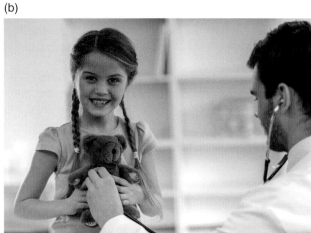

Figure 4.3 Approaching an older child

Adolescents

One might imagine that adolescents would be as simple to examine as adults, but it must be remembered that they also have not reached either emotional, or physical, maturity. While some may be mature and calm, others may be quite uncooperative. Often they are afraid to voice their anxieties, in case they 'look silly'. It is important to remember to reassure this age group, despite their apparent maturity.

Some of these young people will have hidden agendas. It is possible that they should not have been where they were when an accident occurred, or perhaps their depressed conscious level is due to the ingestion of alcohol or drugs. Possibly, they are concealing a pregnancy. Confrontation and humiliation will not be helpful.

Mental health presentations begin to become commoner in this age group and can be very challenging. Self-harm becomes more prevalent than in younger children and somatisation occurs, with physical symptoms presenting instead of more typical mental health symptoms.

Finally, it is important to remember that young people in this group are often extremely shy and every effort must be made to respect their wishes and preserve their modesty. Consider same gender examination if appropriate and where possible, especially for those with particular religious or cultural prohibitions.

4.2 Assessing children: some practical considerations

Trends are more valuable than individual observations, therefore it is important to note the time when each observation was made so the clinical course can be monitored.

Catastrophic haemorrhage (the < C > ABC approach)

> **In the injured child the absolute priority is the control of catastrophic haemorrhage.**

Recognise and treat life-threatening haemorrhage. This ONLY means haemorrhage likely to cause death within minutes.

Limb

Apply an arterial tourniquet. An example is shown in Figure 4.4. The tourniquet should be applied as low as possible to reduce tissue injury. If distal bleeding is not controlled, consider a second tourniquet.

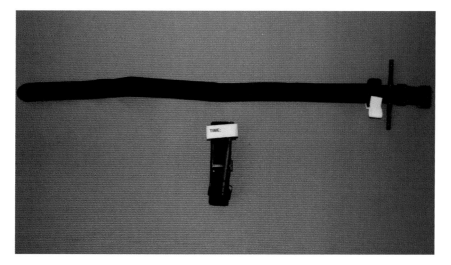

Figure 4.4 Manual arterial tourniquet

If the bleeding is still not controlled, pack the wound with haemostatic impregnated gauze and dressings and apply direct pressure. Transfer to hospital immediately with a pre-alert message.

Be aware that tourniquets are very painful when applied at an effective pressure. Note the time of application and be absolutely certain that the receiving team are aware of their use. Tourniquets should not be applied for more than 60 minutes.

Pelvis

Pelvic fractures can cause exsanguination in children and should be considered a source of catastrophic haemorrhage. A variety of pelvic splints are available, not all of which will fit all children. Whatever you do carry, be familiar with its correct application as this is commonly done badly. Pelvic injuries are suspected by the mechanism of injury, asymmetry, pain, bruising and blood from either the anus, vagina or urethra. If suspected, a splint should be applied as early as possible.

Head, torso and junctional areas

Apply direct pressure continuously with a dressing directly over the wound. Most bleeding can be controlled in this manner.

If this does not control the bleeding, apply a haemostatic dressing as per the manufacturer's specification (this often requires a two-person technique) and reapply the dressings with direct and continuous pressure. Transfer to hospital immediately with a pre-alert message.

4.3 Primary assessment of the airway and breathing

Assessment of the airway

Manual immobilisation of the cervical spine should be implemented immediately if there is a blunt mechanism of trauma consistent with cervical injury or neurological deficit **and** the child is cooperative (it is not indicated in penetrating trauma). The airway should be assessed as below.

> **Assess the position and patency of the airway, and look for the signs and sounds of an obstructed airway.**

Open the airway and:

- Look for the chest rising
- Listen for breathing
- Feel for breath on your cheek
- **If there are no signs of breathing, commence basic life support**

Assessment of breathing

One simple system to use is shown in the following box.

> **RIPPA**
>
> | | |
> |---|---|
> | **R** | Respiratory rate |
> | **I** | Inspection |
> | **P** | Palpation |
> | **P** | Percussion |
> | **A** | Auscultation |

In further assessment of breathing, look for effort of breathing, efficacy of breathing and effect of breathing bearing in mind the effects of respiratory inadequacy on other organs in the child's body.

Effort of breathing

The degree of increase in the effort of breathing allows clinical assessment of the severity of the respiratory problem. It is important to assess the following:

Respiratory rate

Normal resting respiratory rates at differing ages are shown in Table 4.1. The respiratory rate should be counted over 30 seconds to improve the accuracy of the measurement.

Table 4.1 Respiratory rate by age at rest			
Age (years)	Respiratory rate (breaths/min)	Age (years)	Respiratory rate (breaths/min)
Birth to 1 month	25–50	2–7 years	20–30
3 months	25–45	8–11 years	15–25
6–12 months	20–40	12 years to adult	12–24
18 months	20–35		

Rates are higher in infancy and fall with increasing age. Care should be taken in interpreting single measurements: infants can show rates of between 30 and 90 breaths per minute, dependent on their state of activity. Most useful are trends in the measurement as an indicator of improvement or deterioration. At rest, tachypnoea indicates that increased ventilation is needed because of either lung or airway disease, or metabolic acidosis. A slow respiratory rate indicates fatigue, cerebral depression, or a pre-terminal state.

Recession

Intercostal, subcostal, sternal or suprasternal (tracheal tug) recession shows increased effort of breathing. This sign is more easily seen in younger infants as they have a more compliant chest wall. Its presence in older children (i.e. over 6 or 7 years) suggests severe respiratory problems. The degree of recession gives an indication of the severity of respiratory difficulty. Be aware, however, in the child who has become exhausted through increased effort of breathing that recession decreases or is absent.

Inspiratory or expiratory noises

An inspiratory noise while breathing (stridor) is a sign of upper airway, laryngeal or tracheal obstruction. In severe obstruction the stridor may also occur in expiration, but the inspiratory component is usually more pronounced. Wheezing indicates lower airway narrowing and is more pronounced in expiration. A prolonged expiratory phase also indicates lower airway narrowing. The volume of the noise is not always an indicator of severity, as it may disappear in the pre-terminal state.

Grunting

Grunting is produced by exhalation against a partially closed glottis. It is an attempt to generate a positive end-expiratory pressure and to prevent airway collapse at the end of expiration, thereby improving oxygenation. This is a sign of severe respiratory distress and is characteristically seen in infants with pneumonia or pulmonary oedema. It may also be seen with raised intracranial pressure, abdominal distension or peritonism.

Accessory muscle use

The sternomastoid muscle may be used as an accessory respiratory muscle when the effort of breathing is increased. In infants, this is ineffectual and just causes the head to bob up and down with each breath. The presence of head bobbing indicates significant respiratory distress.

Flaring of the nostrils

Flaring of the nostrils is seen especially in infants with respiratory distress.

Gasping

This is a sign of severe hypoxia and may be pre-terminal.

Exceptions

There may be absent or decreased evidence of increased effort of breathing in three circumstances:

1. In the infant or child who has had severe respiratory problems for some time, fatigue may occur and the signs of increased effort of breathing will decrease. ***Exhaustion is a pre-terminal sign***.
2. Children with cerebral depression from raised intracranial pressure, poisoning or encephalopathy will have respiratory inadequacy without increased effort of breathing. The respiratory inadequacy in this case is caused by decreased respiratory drive.
3. Children who have neuromuscular disease (such as spinal muscular atrophy or muscular dystrophy) may present in respiratory failure without increased effort of breathing.

The diagnosis of respiratory failure in such children is made by observing the efficacy of breathing, and looking for other signs of respiratory inadequacy. These are discussed in the text.

Efficacy of breathing

Observation of the degree of chest expansion (or, in infants, abdominal excursion) provides an indication of the amount of air being inspired and expired. Similarly, important information is given by auscultation of the chest. Listen for reduced, asymmetrical or bronchial breath sounds. **A silent chest is an extremely worrying sign.**

Pulse oximetry can be used to measure the arterial oxygen saturation (SpO$_2$). Oximetry in air gives a good indication of the efficacy of breathing by using oxygenation as a surrogate marker of ventilation. A good plethysmographic (pulse) waveform is important to help confirm the accuracy of measurements. In severe shock and hypothermia, there may be poor or absent pulse detection. Measurements are also less accurate when the SpO$_2$ is less than 70%, with motion artefact, and in the presence of carboxyhaemoglobin. To further accurately assess the adequacy of ventilation, some measure of end-tidal carbon dioxide should be obtained. Normal SpO$_2$ in an infant or child at sea level is 97–100%.

Effects of breathing

Heart rate

Hypoxia produces tachycardia in the older infant and child. Anxiety and a fever will also contribute to tachycardia, making this a non-specific sign. **Severe or prolonged hypoxia leads to bradycardia. This is a pre-terminal sign.**

Skin colour

Hypoxia (via catecholamine release) produces vasoconstriction and skin pallor. **Cyanosis is a late and pre-terminal sign of hypoxia** as it usually appears when SpO$_2$ falls to <70%, and only in the absence of anaemia. By the time central cyanosis, marked by a blue tongue and mucosa rather than just blue peripheries, is visible in acute respiratory disease, the patient is close to respiratory arrest. In the anaemic child, cyanosis may never be visible despite profound hypoxia. A few children will be cyanosed because of cyanotic heart disease, but may have adequate oxygen delivery (for them). Their cyanoses will be largely unchanged by oxygen therapy.

Mental status

The hypoxic or hypercapnic child will be agitated and/or drowsy. Over time drowsiness increases and eventually consciousness is lost. A generalised muscular hypotonia also accompanies hypoxic cerebral depression. These extremely useful and important signs are often more difficult to detect in small infants. The parents may say that the infant is just 'not himself'. The clinician must assess the child's state of alertness by gaining eye contact, noting the response to voice and, if necessary, to painful stimuli.

4.4 Primary assessment of the circulation

Recognition of potential circulatory failure

Review the control of catastrophic haemorrhage, checking dressings, tourniquets and pelvic splints before progressing further.

Heart rate

Normal rates are shown in Table 4.2. The heart rate initially increases in shock due to catecholamine release and as compensation for decreased stroke volume. The rate, particularly in small infants, may be extremely high (up to 220 per minute).

Table 4.2 Heart rate by age

Age (years)	Heart rate (beats/min)	Age (years)	Heart rate (beats/min)
Birth to 1 month	120–170	4–5 years	80–135
3 months	115–160	6–7 years	80–130
6–12 months	110–160	8–11 years	70–120
18 months	100–155	12 years	65–115
2 years	100–150	14 years to adult	60–110
3 years	90–140		

An abnormally slow pulse rate, or bradycardia, is defined as less than 60 beats per minute or a rapidly falling heart rate associated with poor systemic perfusion. This is a pre-terminal sign.

Pulse volume

Although blood pressure is maintained until shock is severe, an indication of perfusion can be gained by comparative palpation of both the peripheral and central pulses. Absent peripheral pulses and weak central pulses are serious signs of advanced shock and indicate that hypotension is already present. Bounding pulses may be caused by an increased cardiac output (e.g. septicaemia), an arterio-venous systemic shunt (e.g. patent arterial duct) or hypercapnia. Although it is accepted by some that in adults the various pulse points correlate to certain levels of systolic blood pressure, this does not apply to children; although clearly the presence of a radial pulse indicates that a degree of peripheral perfusion is maintained.

Capillary refill

Following cutaneous pressure on the centre of the sternum (or on a digit in the case of pigmented skin) for 5 seconds, capillary refill should occur within 2–3 seconds. A slower refill time than this can indicate poor skin perfusion. This may be a helpful sign in early septic shock when the child may otherwise be apparently well, with warm peripheries.

The presence of fever does not affect the sensitivity of delayed capillary refill in children with hypovolaemia, but a low ambient temperature reduces its specificity, so the sign should be used with caution in trauma patients who have been in a cold environment.

In children with pigmented skin, the sign is more difficult to assess. In these cases the nail beds are used and, additionally, the sole of the feet in young babies.

The capillary refill should not be used as the only indicator of shock.

Blood pressure

Blood pressure is not routinely taken in children in the pre-hospital emergency setting, as it is of limited use in acute management. If it is taken, it requires the correct sized cuff for the child. **Measured hypotension is considered a pre-terminal sign**.

Effects of circulatory inadequacy on other organs

Respiratory system

A rapid respiration rate with an increased tidal volume, *but without recession*, is caused by the oxygen demand and metabolic acidosis resulting from circulatory failure. Increased respiratory rate is an early and often overlooked sign of an unwell child.

Skin

Mottled, cold, pale skin peripherally indicates poor perfusion. A line of coldness may be felt to move centrally as circulatory failure progresses. Limb temperature may improve as resuscitation successfully progresses.

Mental status

Agitation and then drowsiness leading to unconsciousness are characteristic of circulatory failure. These signs are caused by poor cerebral perfusion and hypoxia in an infant. Parents may report abnormal behaviour such as being irritable, inconsolable or sleepier than usual.

Renal function

A history of reduced wet nappies or urine production should be sought.

Cardiac failure

The following features suggest a cardiac cause of respiratory inadequacy:

- Cyanosis, not correcting with oxygen therapy
- Tachycardia out of proportion to respiratory difficulty
- Raised jugular venous pressure
- Gallop rhythm/murmur
- Enlarged liver
- Absent femoral pulses

Note: not all signs will be present in all patients.

4.5 Primary assessment of disability

Recognition of potential central neurological failure

Neurological assessment should only be performed after catastrophic haemorrhage (<C>), airway (A), breathing (B) and circulation (C) have been assessed and treated. There are no neurological problems that take priority over ABC.

Both respiratory and circulatory failure will have central neurological effects. Conversely, some conditions with direct central neurological effects (such as meningitis, raised intracranial pressure from trauma and status epilepticus) may also have respiratory and circulatory consequences.

As part of the assessment of disability it is important to **check the blood sugar** – this can either be done at this point or earlier if cannulating the child as part of the emergency management of circulatory problems.

Conscious level

A rapid assessment of conscious level can be made by assigning the patient to one of the categories shown in the box. When using the AVPU also note the pupillary assessment.

A	ALERT
V	responds to VOICE
P	responds only to PAIN
U	UNRESPONSIVE to all stimuli

If the child does not respond to voice, it is important that assessment is made of the response to pain. The painful central stimulus can be delivered by a firm squeeze to the trapezius. Supraorbital pressure is often used but this may distress parents. A child who is unresponsive or who only responds to pain has a significant degree of coma.

AVPU/GCS

If the child does not respond to voice, then a painful stimulus is needed. If the child responds to pain, note what the eyes and limbs did and what sounds or words were uttered, rather than simply categorising the child as 'P'. Simple descriptions that will form the basis of a subsequent formal Glasgow Coma Score (GCS), such as 'opening eyes to pain' or 'localising to pain' are much more informative than 'P' alone. A child who does not open his/her eyes to pain, utters no sounds and extends his limbs has a GCS of 4 and is likely to need prompt airway protection. A child who opens his/her eyes to pain, shouts recognisable words inappropriately and localises to the stimulus has a GCS of 10 and is at much less immediate risk. Both are classified as 'P'.

Posture

Many children who are suffering from a serious illness in any system are hypotonic (floppy). Stiff posturing, such as that shown by decorticate (flexed arms, extended legs) or decerebrate (extended arms, extended legs) children, is a sign of serious brain dysfunction (Figure 4.5).

(a)   (b)

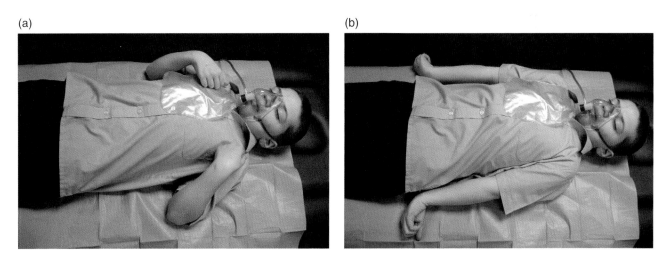

Figure 4.5 (a) Decorticate posturing, and (b) decerebrate posturing

These postures can be mistaken for the tonic phase of a convulsion.

Alternatively, a painful stimulus may be necessary to elicit these postures. Severe extension of the neck due to upper airway obstruction can mimic the opisthotonus that occurs with meningeal irritation. A stiff neck and full fontanelle in infants are signs that suggest meningitis.

Pupils

Drugs, hypoxia, hypovolaemia, intracranial pressure and cerebral lesions have effects on pupil size and reactions. However, the most important pupillary signs are dilatation, unreactivity and inequality, which indicate possible serious intracranial pathology.

Respiratory effects of central neurological failure

There are several recognisable breathing pattern abnormalities with raised intracranial pressure. However, they are often changeable and may vary from hyperventilation to agonal breathing to apnoea. The presence of any abnormal respiratory pattern in a patient with coma suggests mid- or brain stem dysfunction.

Circulatory effects of central neurological failure

Systemic hypertension with sinus bradycardia (Cushing's response) indicates compression of the brain stem caused by raised intracranial pressure. **This is a late and pre-terminal sign.**

4.6 Assessment of exposure

Exposure of the seriously ill child by removing clothing will enable examination for markers of illness that will help guide specific emergency treatment.

Temperature

A fever suggests an infection as the cause of the illness, but may also be the result of prolonged convulsions or shivering. In young infants, infection may present with a low body temperature.

Rash

Examination is made for rashes, such as urticaria in allergic reactions, purpura, petechiae and bruising in septicaemia and child abuse, or maculo-papular and erythematous rashes in allergic reactions and some forms of sepsis.

The box shows a summary for the rapid clinical assessment of an infant or child.

Summary: the rapid clinical assessment of an infant or child

Catastrophic haemorrhage **< C>**
    Visible peripheral haemorrhage
    Suspected pelvic injury
Airway and **B**reathing
    Effort of breathing
    Respiratory rate/rhythm
    Stridor/wheeze
    Equality of chest movements
    Auscultation
    Skin colour
Circulation
    Heart rate
    Pulse volume
    Capillary refill
    Skin temperature
    Reduced urine output with fewer wet nappies than usual
Disability
    Mental status/conscious level (AVPU or GCS)
    Posture
    Pupils
    Check blood sugar
Exposure
    Temperature
    Rash and bruising

The whole assessment should take less than a minute. Once airway (A), breathing (B) and circulation (C) are clearly recognised as being stable or have been stabilised, then definitive management of the underlying condition can proceed. During definitive management reassessment of ABCD at frequent intervals will be necessary to assess progress and detect deterioration.

Injury

Consideration of injury is particularly important in the non-ambulatory child or on other occasions when non-accidental injury is suspected.

Reassessment

Single observations on respiratory and heart rates, degree of recession, blood pressure, conscious level, pupils, etc. are useful, but much more information can be gained by frequent, repeated observations to detect a trend in the patient's condition.

4.7 Primary assessment and resuscitation

In a severely ill or injured child, the rapid examination of vital functions is combined with immediate necessary resuscitation. The assessment is done following the approach discussed in Sections 4.1–4.5 following the < C > ABC approach. This primary assessment and any necessary resuscitation must be completed before the more detailed secondary assessment is performed.

Catastrophic haemorrhage

See Section 4.2.

Airway

Primary assessment

See Section 4.3.

Resuscitation

- If the airway is not patent, then this can be secured by:
  - a chin lift or jaw thrust – airway opening manoeuvres
  - the use of an airway adjunct, e.g. an oro- or nasopharyngeal airway
  - a supraglottic airway device (SAD) or, exceptionally, tracheal intubation by trained and experienced rescuers
- **Reassess the airway after any airway opening manoeuvres**

Breathing

Primary assessment

See Section 4.3.

A patent airway does not ensure adequate ventilation. The latter requires an intact respiratory centre and adequate pulmonary function, augmented by coordinated movement of the diaphragm and chest wall.

Resuscitation

- Give high-flow oxygen through a non-rebreathing mask with a reservoir bag to any child with respiratory difficulty or hypoxia at a sufficient flow rate to keep the reservoir bag distended (or 15 l/min if supplies are not limited)
- In the child with inadequate breathing, this should be supported with bag–valve–mask ventilation. Adjuncts may be required, such as an oro- or nasopharyngeal airway, and an SAD may be considered

Circulation

See Section 4.4.

Primary assessment

The assessment of circulation has been described. *It is more difficult to assess than breathing and individual measurements must not be overinterpreted.* An overall 'picture' of all the parameters and any possible confounding factors, along with underlying causes, should always be considered.

Resuscitation

- Give high-flow oxygen to every child with an inadequate circulation (shock). This will be through either a non-rebreathing mask with a reservoir bag, or via bag-valve-mask, or SAD for inadequate breathing or airway control
- In children with suspected sepsis, venous or intraosseous access should be gained and an immediate infusion of crystalloid (usually 0.9% saline) given at a dose of 10 ml/kg (this can be repeated immediately if there is no clinical improvement). More than 40 ml/kg should not usually be necessary and great care should be given to continuously monitor the response if this is done. If the child deteriorates, or develops increasing breathlessness, the fluid should be stopped

Reassessment of < C > ABC after each bolus (or during it, if possible, as well) is essential and the fluid should be repeated if needed.

In trauma, boluses should be of 5 ml/kg each with reassessment after each bolus. The boluses should be repeated until there is a substantial improvement in the circulatory status of the child **towards** normal, using the presence of a radial pulse as a guide. It may not be possible to normalise all vital signs for reasons other than hypovolaemia (e.g. a tachycardia may be caused by pain or anxiety). It is important not to overfill children with serious trauma. Fluids administered must be accurately documented and a detailed handover given at the hospital.

Disability (neurological evaluation)

Primary assessment

See Section 4.5.

Both hypoxia and shock can cause a decrease in conscious level. *Any problem with ABC must be addressed before assuming that a decrease in conscious level is due to a primary neurological problem.* The rapid assessment of central neurological failure has been described. Remember any patient with a decreased conscious level or convulsions must have an initial glucose stick test performed.

Resuscitation

Consider early onward referral to definitively stabilise the airway (intubation) in any child with a conscious level recorded as 'P' or 'U' (only responding to painful stimuli or unresponsive), unless competent to do this – considerable experience in in-hospital paediatric anaesthesia is recommended. Ensure the airway is kept as clear as possible (if necessary using adjuncts if the patient does not have a gag reflex) until this is done.

Treat hypoglycaemia with a bolus of glucose (2 ml/kg of 10% glucose), followed by regular monitoring of the blood sugar and repeat doses if needed, or by an intravenous infusion of glucose if available.

Buccal midazolam or rectal diazepam followed, if needed, by intravenous lorazepam should initially be given for fits lasting more than 5 minutes (see Convulsions section, Chapter 5).

Manage raised intracranial pressure, if present (see Coma management section, Chapter 5).

CHAPTER 5

Immediate management of the seriously ill child

Learning outcomes

After reading this chapter, you will be able to:
- Describe how to recognise airway, breathing, circulation and neurological emergencies in children
- Describe the emergency treatment required for airway, breathing, circulation and neurological emergencies in children

---

5.1 Introduction

Serious illness in children is relatively rare. The majority of children seen within the healthcare system are presenting with self-limiting illness, which can be worrying and stressful to the child's parents but not life threatening. However, in young children and infants it can be difficult to distinguish between a serious infection and a self-limiting viral illness. For example, where the only sign that an infant is unwell is a subtle change in their sleeping or eating patterns, the role of the healthcare provider is to distinguish between life-threatening presentations and self-limiting illness. This may be difficult at times, and demands history taking, thorough examination and clinical experience.

General rules

- Always take a history
- Always carry out a full set of observations including respiratory rate, heart rate, temperature and capillary refill. Blood pressure can be taken if it will alter management and the correctly sized cuff is available
- The younger the child, the lower the threshold for seeking specialist paediatric advice
- Always take a blood sugar for children and infants who have an altered level of consciousness or a history of a convulsion
- Regular reassessment is important, especially if the transfer is prolonged or in a remote setting
- If concerned, a period of observation within an appropriate environment is always useful and should be encouraged
- Always involve the parents and their child in decision making
- If leaving the child at home, always provide clear, written safety advice, highlighting the red flags for seeking immediate advice and where to get that advice

---

The main symptoms likely to be encountered in a pre-hospital emergency are discussed here. There is a brief discussion followed by an algorithm. It is important to use the structured approach in the assessment of the ill child to ensure that the more subtle signs are recognised.

Pre-Hospital Paediatric Life Support: A Practical Approach to Emergencies, Third Edition. Edited by Alan Charters, Hal Maxwell and Paul Reavley.
© 2017 John Wiley & Sons Ltd. Published 2017 by John Wiley & Sons Ltd.

5.2 Airway difficulties

Background

A summary of sudden causes of airway difficulties is given in Table 5.1.

Table 5.1 Sudden causes of airway difficulties

Incidence (UK)	Diagnosis	Clinical features
Very common	Croup – viral laryngotracheitis	Coryzal, barking cough, mild fever, hoarse voice, stridor
Common	Croup – recurrent or spasmodic croup	Sudden onset, recurrent, history of atopy
Uncommon	Laryngeal foreign body	Sudden onset, history of choking
Rare	Epiglottitis	Drooling, muffled voice, septic appearance
	Croup – bacterial tracheitis	Harsh cough, chest pain, septic appearance
	Trauma	Neck swelling, crepitus or bruising
	Retropharyngeal abscess	Drooling, septic appearance
	Inhalation of hot gases	Facial burns, peri-oral soot
	Angioneurotic oedema	Itching, facial swelling, urticarial rash
	Diphtheria	Travel to endemic area, unimmunised

What to look for

In general, added inspiratory sounds indicate obstruction in the upper airway. Whereas added expiratory sounds (wheeze) indicate problems in the lower airway.

- If 'bubbly' noises are heard, the airway is full of secretions requiring clearance. This also suggests that the child is either very fatigued or has a depressed conscious level and cannot clear the secretions himself, or herself, by coughing
- If stertorous (snoring) respiratory noises are heard, consider partial obstruction of the airway due to a depressed conscious level or a 'high up' obstruction such as a peri-tonsillar abscess (quinsy)
- If there is a harsh stridor associated with a barking cough, upper airway obstruction due to croup should be suspected
- With a very sudden onset, no prodromal symptoms and a history suggestive of inhalation, consider a laryngeal foreign body
- The abnormal speech heard with retropharyngeal abscess is sometimes described as sounding as if the person 'has a hot potato in their mouth'

> In the child with a compromised but functioning airway, an important principle in all cases is to avoid worsening the situation by upsetting the child. Crying and struggling may quickly convert a partially obstructed airway into a completely obstructed one. Administration of oxygen or nebulised adrenaline may require skill. Parents' help should be enlisted. The throat should be examined very carefully and not at all if epiglottitis is suspected.

Specific conditions

Croup

Croup is defined as an acute clinical syndrome with inspiratory stridor, a barking cough, hoarseness and variable degrees of respiratory distress. This definition embraces several distinct disorders. Acute viral laryngotracheobronchitis (viral croup) is the commonest form of croup and accounts for over 95% of laryngotracheal infections. The peak incidence of viral croup is in the second year of life and most hospital admissions are in children aged between 6 months and 5 years. Many children have stridor and a mild fever (<38.5 °C), with severity varying from no respiratory difficulty to a few (less than 5%, usually aged under 3 years) who develop life-threatening respiratory obstruction.

Management

Oral dexamethasone has been shown to improve symptoms of croup within as short a time as 45 minutes. If the oral solution is not available, the IV preparation can be used orally. Nebulised budesonide is also very effective, but may upset the child and takes longer to administer.

The dose of oral dexamethasone in croup is 0.15 mg/kg, repeated at 12 hours if required.

The dose of nebulised budesonide is 2 mg.

Practitioners carrying prednisolone, rather than dexamethasone, are advised as follows: where it is thought there could be benefit in pre-hospital administration (e.g. during a prolonged retrieval), and dexamethasone is not available, soluble prednisolone can be given at 2 mg/kg up to 40 mg.

If the child is developing signs of severe respiratory failure, nebulised adrenaline can be given and is likely to give almost immediate significant improvement for up to 2 hours. Give 0.4 ml/kg of 1/1000 adrenaline solution (maximum 5 ml) via a nebuliser, and repeat after 30 minutes if required.

Foreign body

Do not try to remove a foreign body if the child is conscious – a partial obstruction can become a total obstruction (see Section 7.4).

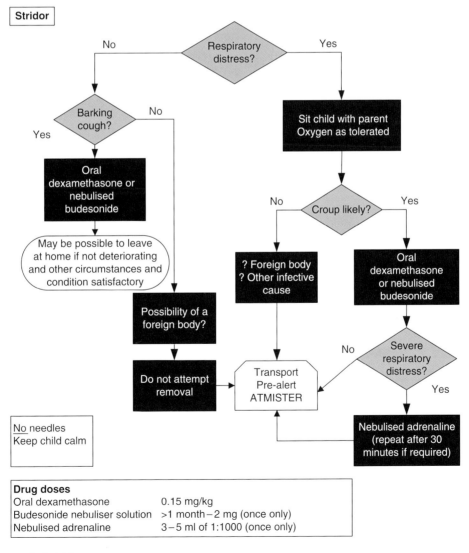

Figure 5.1 Management of stridor

5.3 Breathing

Summary of breathing problems

Disorders affecting the lungs	Asthma
	Viral-induced wheeze
	Bronchiolitis
	Pneumonia
	Pulmonary oedema
Disorders around the lungs	Pneumothorax
	Empyema
	Haemothorax
	Rib fractures
Disorders of the respiratory muscle	Neuromuscular disorders
Disorders below the diaphragm	Peritonitis
	Abdominal distension (gastric insufflation, bowel obstruction)
Increased respiratory drive	Metabolic acidosis (e.g. diabetic ketoacidosis)
	Shock
	Poisoning
	Anxiety/hyperventilation
Decreased respiratory drive	Coma
	Convulsions
	Raised intracranial pressure
	Poisoning

There are a wide range of problems that may cause breathing difficulties in children. Disorders of the respiratory tract are the commonest cause of illness in children. They are the most frequent reason for children to be seen by their general practitioner and account for 40% of acute hospital admissions. However, there are disorders outside the respiratory tract that can cause breathing compromise such as cardiac disease, poisoning and metabolic disorders.

Causes of breathing difficulties in children

Background

Bronchiolitis occurs in 10% of all infants and 2–3% are admitted to hospital with the disease each year. Ninety per cent of patients are aged 1–9 months – it is rare after 1 year of age. Respiratory syncytial virus is the pathogen in 60–70% of cases, the remainder of cases being caused by other respiratory viruses such as parainfluenza, influenza and adenoviruses.

Fever and a clear nasal discharge precede a dry cough and increasing breathlessness. Wheezing is often, but not always, present. Feeding difficulty associated with increasing dyspnoea and resulting in poor intake and dehydration is often the reason for admission to hospital, with hypoxia or respiratory distress being the others. Recurrent apnoea is a serious and potentially fatal complication and is seen particularly in infants born prematurely.

What to look for

Bronchiolitis signs

Tachypnoea	50–100 breaths/min
Recession	Subcostal and intercostal
Cough	Sharp, dry
Hyperinflation of the chest	Sternum prominent, liver depressed
Tachycardia	140–200 beats/min
Crackles	Fine end-inspiratory
Wheeze	High-pitched expiratory > inspiratory
Colour	Cyanosis or pallor
Breathing pattern	Irregular breathing/recurrent apnoea

Assess ABC:

- Ensure that the airway is patent and clear; use of a Yankauer suction catheter applied to the nares can help to ensure that the nose and nasopharynx are cleared, which can have a significant impact on an infant's respiratory distress
- Give a high concentration of oxygen via a mask with reservoir bag to maintain oxygen saturations at >94%
- Monitor for apnoea/hypoventilation especially in those <2 months old:
  - SpO_2
  - respiratory frequency/apnoea
- Bronchodilators, steroids and antibiotics are of no proven value

Asthma

Background

Asthma affects over 1.1 million children in the UK. Asthma attacks hospitalise a child every 8 minutes; 185 children are admitted to hospital because of asthma attacks every day in the UK (Asthma UK).

What to look for

It can be difficult to assess the *severity* of an acute exacerbation of asthma. Clinical signs correlate poorly with the severity of airway obstruction. Some children with acute severe asthma do not appear distressed, and young children with severe asthma are especially difficult to assess.

Historical features associated with more severe or life-threatening airway obstruction include:

- A long duration of symptoms and symptoms of regular nocturnal awakening
- A poor response to treatment already given in this episode
- A severe course of previous attacks, including the use of intravenous therapy, and those who have required admission to an intensive care unit

Two characteristic levels are described to indicate the appearance of asthmatic children at the most severe end of the spectrum. These are **severe** and **life-threatening** asthma (Table 5.2).

Table 5.2 Features of moderate, acute severe and life-threatening asthma		
Moderate asthma	**Acute severe asthma**	**Life-threatening asthma**
$SpO_2 \geq 92\%$	Too breathless to feed or talk	Exhaustion Poor respiratory effort
No clinical features of severe or life-threatening attack	Recession/use of accessory muscles	Silent chest

Peak flow >50% of best/predicted	Respiratory rate:
	    >30/min (>5 years)
	    >50/min (2–5 years)
		$SpO_2 < 92\%$ in air/cyanosis
		Peak flow <33% of best/predicted
		Hypotension

	Pulse rate:
	    >120 beats/min (>5 years)
	    >130 beats/min (2–5 years)
		Conscious level depressed/agitated

	Peak flow 33–50% of best/predicted	CONSIDER WHETHER THIS COULD BE ANAPHYLAXIS

Age 2–5 years

ASSESS ASTHMA SEVERITY

Moderate asthma	Severe asthma	Life-threatening asthma
▪ $SpO_2 \geq 92\%$	▪ $SpO_2 < 92\%$	$SpO_2 < 92\%$ plus any of:
▪ Able to talk	▪ Too breathless to talk	▪ Silent chest
▪ Heart rate ≤ 140/min	▪ Heart rate > 140/min	▪ Poor respiratory effort
▪ Respiratory rate ≤ 40/min	▪ Respiratory rate > 40/min	▪ Agitation
	▪ Use of accessory neck muscles	▪ Altered consciousness
		▪ Cyanosis

▪ β_2 agonist 2–10 puffs via spacer and face mask (given one puff at a time inhaled separately using tidal breathing)
 	
▪ Give one puff of β_2 agonist every 30–60 seconds up to 10 puffs according to response
 	
▪ Consider soluble prednisolone 20 mg
	▪ Oxygen via face mask
	
	▪ 10 puffs of β_2 agonist or nebulised salbutamol 2.5 mg
	
	▪ Soluble prednisolone 20 mg
	
	Assess response to treatment 15 min after β_2 agonist
		▪ Oxygen via face mask
		
		▪ Nebulise every 20 min with:
		  - salbutamol 2.5 mg
		    +
		  - ipratropium 0.25 mg
		
		▪ Soluble prednisolone 20 mg or IV hydrocortisone 50 mg

IF POOR RESPONSE ARRANGE ADMISSION	**IF POOR RESPONSE REPEAT β_2 AGONIST AND ARRANGE ADMISSION**	**REPEAT β_2 AGONIST VIA OXYGEN-DRIVEN NEBULISER WHILST ARRANGING IMMEDIATE HOSPITAL ADMISSION**

GOOD RESPONSE

▪ Continue β_2 agonist via spacer or nebuliser, as needed but not exceeding 4 hourly

▪ **If symptoms are not controlled repeat β_2 agonist and refer to hospital**

▪ Continue prednisolone for up to 3 days

▪ Arrange follow-up clinic visit

POOR RESPONSE

▪ Stay with patient until ambulance arrives

▪ Send written assessment and referral details

▪ Repeat β_2 agonist via oxygen-driven nebuliser in ambulance

---

LOWER THRESHOLD FOR ADMISSION IF:

▪ Attack in late afternoon or at night

▪ Recent hospital admission or previous severe attack

▪ Concern over social circumstances or ability to cope at home

NB: If a patient has signs and symptoms across categories, always treat according to their most severe features

Figure 5.2 Management of acute asthma in children in general practice: (a) children aged 2–5 years, (b) children aged >5 years.
PEF, peak expiratory flow. British Thoracic Society; Scottish Intercollegiate Guidelines Network. British guideline on the management of asthma. *Thorax* 2014 Nov;69(Suppl. 1):1–192. Epub 2014 Oct 16. Reproduced with permission of BMJ Publishing Group Ltd

Age > 5 years

ASSESS ASTHMA SEVERITY

Moderate asthma

- $SpO_2 \geq 92\%$
- PEF ≥ 50% best or predicted
- Able to talk
- Heart rate ≤ 125/min
- Respiratory rate ≤ 30/min

Severe asthma

- $SpO_2 < 92\%$
- PEF 33–50% best or predicted
- Too breathless to talk
- Heart rate > 125/min
- Respiratory rate > 30/min
- Use of accessory neck muscles

Life-threatening asthma

$SpO_2 < 92\%$ plus any of:

- PEF < 33% best or predicted
- Silent chest
- Poor respiratory effort
- Agitation
- Altered consciousness
- Cyanosis

▼

- β_2 agonist 2–10 puffs via spacer and mouthpiece (given one puff at a time inhaled separately using tidal breathing).
- Give one puff of β_2 agonist every 30–60 seconds up to 10 puffs according to response.
- Consider soluble prednisolone 30–40 mg

▼

- Oxygen via face mask
- 10 puffs of β_2 agonist or nebulised salbutamol 5 mg
- Soluble prednisolone 30–40 mg

Assess response to treatment 15 min after β_2 agonist

▼

- Oxygen via face mask
- Nebulise every 20 min with:
  - salbutamol 5 mg
    +
  - ipratropium 0.25 mg
- Soluble prednisolone 30–40 mg
  or
  IV hydrocortisone 100 mg

▼ ▼ ▼

IF POOR RESPONSE ARRANGE ADMISSION

IF POOR RESPONSE REPEAT β_2 AGONIST AND ARRANGE ADMISSION

REPEAT β_2 AGONIST VIA OXYGEN-DRIVEN NEBULISER WHILST ARRANGING IMMEDIATE HOSPITAL ADMISSION

GOOD RESPONSE

- Continue β_2 agonist via spacer or nebuliser, as needed but not exceeding 4 hourly
- **If symptoms are not controlled repeat β_2 agonist and refer to hospital**
- Continue prednisolone for up to 3 days
- Arrange follow-up clinic visit

POOR RESPONSE

- Stay with patient until ambulance arrives
- Send written assessment and referral details
- Repeat β_2 agonist via oxygen-driven nebuliser in ambulance

LOWER THRESHOLD FOR ADMISSION IF:

- Attack in late afternoon or at night
- Recent hospital admission or previous severe attack
- Concern over social circumstances or ability to cope at home

NB: If a patient has signs and symptoms across categories, always treat according to their most severe features

Figure 5.2 (*Continued*)

After resuscitation, and before progressing to specific treatment for acute asthma in any setting, it is essential to assess accurately the severity of the child's condition. The following clinical signs should be recorded regularly, e.g. every 30 minutes, or before and after each dose of bronchodilator:

- Heart rate
- Respiratory rate and degree of recession
- Use of accessory muscles of respiration
- Degree of agitation and conscious level
- SpO_2
- Peak flow – this should only be done in children over the age of 6 who are not distressed

More intensive in-patient treatment is likely to be needed for children with an SpO_2 of <92% on air after initial bronchodilator treatment.

Management (Figure 5.2)

Assess ABC.

- Give high-flow oxygen via a face mask with a reservoir bag
- Attach pulse oximeter; always aim to keep $SpO_2 > 92\%$
- Give a β-2 agonist, such as salbutamol:
  - in those with mild to moderate asthma and maintaining $SpO_2 > 92\%$ in air, use pressurised aerosol 2–10 sprays as required via a valved holding chamber (spacer) with a mouthpiece or tightly fitting face mask. Children with mild to moderate asthma are less likely to have tachycardia and hypoxia if given β-2 agonists via a pressurised aerosol and spacer. Children aged <3 years are likely to require a face mask connected to the mouthpiece of a spacer for successful drug delivery. Inhalers should be sprayed into the spacer in individual puffs and inhaled immediately by tidal breathing
  - in those with severe asthma, initiate treatment with either 10 puffs of salbutamol via a spacer or 2.5–5 mg salbutamol via a nebuliser
  - in life-threatening asthma, or when oxygen is needed, use nebulised salbutamol 2.5 mg (<5 years) or 5 mg (>5 years) (with ipratropium bromide) with oxygen at a flow of 4–6 l/min in order to provide small enough particle sizes. Higher flows may be used, but more of the nebulised drug may be lost from the face mask
  - give oral prednisolone 1–2 mg/kg (max. 40 mg) or, if vomiting, IV hydrocortisone 4 mg/kg (max. 200 mg)
- If the child is vomiting and becomes distressed by the thought of cannulation consider waiting until in hospital for the steroids to be given
- If breathing fails to improve in severe asthma in those receiving nebulised salbutamol, add ipratropium bromide 250 micrograms in the same nebuliser. This may be given every 20–30 minutes initially, reducing the dose as improvement occurs. In severe asthma, the salbutamol nebulisers should be continuous, as breaks between them can lead to rebound of symptoms
- Consider whether this could be anaphylaxis. If the child continues to deteriorate despite salbutamol and ipratropium, treat with adrenaline as for anaphylaxis. Never use adrenaline without the child being on oxygen as it can increase the ventilation:perfusion mismatch

5.4 Shock

Shock results from an acute failure of circulatory function. Inadequate amounts of nutrients, especially oxygen, are delivered to body tissues and there is inadequate removal of tissue waste products. Other than underlying illnesses, age-dependent maturation of different organ systems and the body's defence mechanisms define the response to shock.

Shock is a progressive state which can be divided in phases. Although artificial, this division is useful because each phase has characteristic clinical manifestations and outcomes.

Compensated shock

In this early phase, physiological compensatory mechanisms maintain vital (e.g. brain and heart) organ perfusion.

Uncompensated shock

If shock is unrecognised or untreated in the early stage, it progresses further and the compensatory mechanisms fail to support the circulatory system. Poorly perfused tissues and organs can no longer sustain aerobic metabolism and comparatively inefficient anaerobic metabolism becomes their major source of energy production. During this stage the effects of shock can be reversed with correct resuscitation.

Irreversible shock

If the shock continues untreated, it progresses to an irreversible stage where the cellular damage cannot be reversed even if cardiovascular function is restored to adequate levels. Despite haemodynamic correction, multiple organ failure and death occurs.

Examples of types of shock are listed in the box.

Types of shock

Hypovolaemic	Haemorrhage
	Gastrointestinal (GI) loss
	'Third spacing' GI obstruction, intussusception, volvulus
	Burns
Distributive	Sepsis
	Anaphylaxis
	Vasodilating drugs
	Spinal cord injury
Cardiogenic	Arrhythmias
	Cardiomyopathy
	Heart failure (cardiomyopathy, myocarditis)
	Valvular disease
Obstructive	Congenital cardiac (coarctation, aortic stenosis)
	Tension/haemopneumothorax
	Cardiac tamponade
	Pulmonary embolism
Dissociative	Profound anaemia
	Poisoning, e.g. cyanide
	Methaemoglobinaemia

What to look for

Perform a structured <C>ABCDE assessment to identify and treat life-threatening issues. Remember to adequately expose the child. Exposure may demonstrate rashes associated with meningococcal sepsis or anaphylaxis.

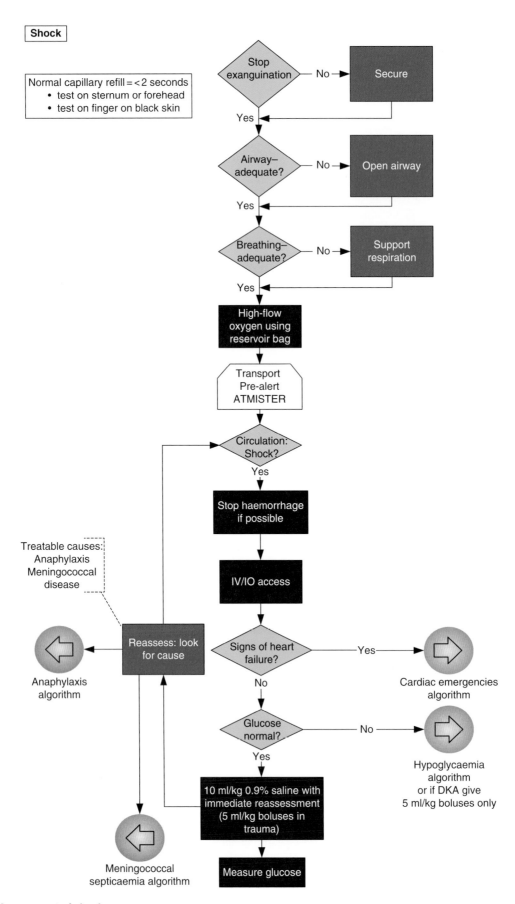

Figure 5.3 Management of shock

Management (Figure 5.3)

- Maintain a patent airway
- All children in shock should receive high-flow oxygen through a face mask with reservoir
- Support breathing as required
- Gain good peripheral venous access. If this is not achieved rapidly, insert an intraosseous line. Give 10 ml/kg rapid bolus of crystalloid to all patients with signs of shock, reassess and repeat to effect, 5 ml/kg in trauma and DKA
- Check blood glucose level and correct if low
- Treat underlying cause. If unclear, treat empirically with antibiotics as per local protocols
- Reassess < C > ABCDE and repeat fluids as needed to improve circulation

Anaphylaxis

Background

Anaphylaxis is a potentially life-threatening, immunologically mediated reaction to ingested, inhaled or topical substances, which may present as either shock and/or respiratory distress.

What to look for

Table 5.3 lists the signs and symptoms to look for.

Table 5.3 Signs and symptoms of allergic and anaphylactic reactions		
	Symptoms	**Signs**
Allergic reactions	Burning sensation in mouth, itching of lips, mouth and throat, coughing, feeling of warmth, nausea, abdominal pain, loose bowel motions, sweating	Urticarial rash, angio-oedema, conjunctivitis
Anaphylaxis	Difficulty breathing, noisy breathing, cyanosis, agitation, collapse	Wheeze, stridor, tachycardia with hypotension, poor pulse volume and pallor, respiratory arrest or cardiac arrest

Management (Figure 5.4)

The management of anaphylactic shock requires airway management, administration of adrenaline and aggressive fluid resuscitation:

- High-flow oxygen via a non-rebreathing mask
- Intramuscular adrenaline: either 10 micrograms/kg; *or* 150 micrograms <6 years, 300 micrograms 6–12 years, or 500 micrograms >12 years; repeated as necessary every 5 minutes until improved. If an Epipen/Anapen or similar is used, the following doses should be administered: age <6 years, one Epipen junior (150 micrograms); age 6–12 years, one Epipen (300 micrograms)
- Nebulised adrenaline 3–5 ml of 1:1000, as for croup (if severe stridor present)
- Nebulised bronchodilator as for asthma

Adrenaline is always given intramuscularly for anaphylaxis, unless cardiac arrest is present – in these cases give via the intravenous or intraosseous route and follow the relevant cardiac arrest protocol.

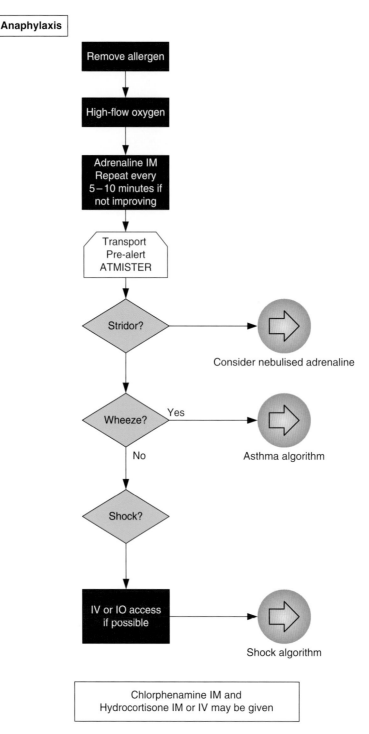

Figure 5.4 Management of anaphylaxis

Septic shock

Background

The incidence of septic shock varies with age and is highest in infants. It carries significant mortality and morbidity. Septic shock is a combination of several factors contributing to the shock. These include: (i) hypovolaemia (fever, often associated diarrhoea, vomiting and anorexia, together with alterations in capillary permeability leading to capillary leakage); (ii) cardiogenic elements (impaired cardiac function due to hypovolaemia and direct myocardial suppressive factors from infecting organisms and the host inflammatory response); (iii) distributive elements (alterations in vascular tone with vasoconstriction in some vascular beds and vasodilatation in others); and (iv) dissociative elements (there is a non-specific sepsis-induced mitochondrial dysfunction impairing cellular oxygen utilisation). Septic shock is defined as sepsis with cardiovascular organ dysfunction.

What to look for

A cardinal sign of meningococcal septicaemia is a purpuric rash in an ill child. At the onset, however, the rash may be absent, or mistaken for more innocent viral rashes such as petechiae, and a careful search should be made for purpura in any unwell child. In about 15% of patients with meningococcal septicaemia, a blanching erythematous rash replaces or precedes a purpuric one, and in 7% of cases no rash occurs.

In toxic shock syndrome, the initial clinical picture includes a high fever, headache, confusion, conjunctival and mucosal hyperaemia (reddening), scarlatiniform rash, subcutaneous oedema, vomiting and watery diarrhoea.

Management

Reassess ABC and support as necessary. The management of meningococcal septicaemia is shown in Figure 5.5.

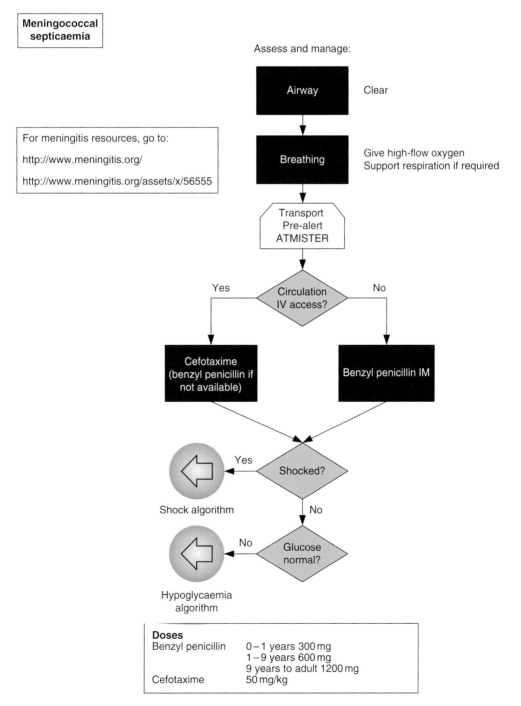

Figure 5.5 Management of meningococcal septicaemia

- Give oxygen to maintain saturations of >95%
- Give a further fluid bolus of 10 ml/kg 0.9% saline if required
- Administer an antibiotic (benzyl penicillin is still recommended outside hospital for meningococcal septicaemia). Cefotaxime can be used if available and there is intravenous or intraosseous access. Ceftriaxone can also be used other than in premature neonates with a corrected gestational age of <41 weeks or in infants less than 1 month old. (See National Institute for Health and Care Excellence (2010) *CG102 Meningitis (bacterial) and meningococcal septicaemia in under 16 s: recognition, diagnosis and management.* Manchester: NICE. Available from www.nice.org.uk/CG102; last accessed February 2017)
- Arrange urgent onward care/transport immediately
- Monitor the Glasgow Coma Scale score – many children with meningococcal disease have an associated meningitis
- If there are signs of raised intracranial pressure (ICP) nurse the patient 30° head up and with the head in the midline. Ensure blood sugar remains normal and blood pressure is maintained if care is prolonged

Coma

Background

The conscious level may be altered by disease, injury or intoxication. As a result of variability in the definition of words describing the degree of coma, the Child's Glasgow Coma Scale (see Table 5.4) has been adopted as a measure of consciousness and, more importantly, as an aid to communication between carers. Ninety-five per cent of coma is caused by metabolic insult, including hypoxia and ischaemia, and 5% from structural causes.

Examples of disorders causing coma in children

Hypoxic ischaemic brain injury following respiratory or circulatory failure
Seizures
Trauma
Intracranial haemorrhage
Cerebral oedema
Meningitis
Encephalitis
Cerebral and extracerebral abscesses
Malaria
Intoxication/drugs
Metabolic causes: renal or hepatic failure, hypo- or hypernatraemia, hypoglycaemia, hypothermia, hypercapnia, inherited metabolic disease
Cerebral tumour
Hydrocephalus, including blocked intraventricular shunts

What to look for

- Abnormal cry
- Mental status/conscious level (AVPU initially, then Glasgow Coma Scale score (Table 5.4) when time allows later)
- Pupillary size and reaction
- Posture: decorticate or decerebrate posturing in a previously normal child should suggest raised ICP
- Neck stiffness in a child
- Full fontanelle in an infant
- The presence of convulsive movements should be sought: these may be subtle

There should be a specific assessment for raised ICP. There are very few absolute signs of raised ICP – these being papilloedema, a bulging fontanelle and the absence of venous pulsation in retinal vessels. All three signs are often absent in acutely raised ICP.

In particular, look for causes that can be easily treated or need very urgent treatment. The big three (after hypoxia/hypotension, which will be picked up and treated in the assessment and management of breathing and circulation) are:

- Hypoglycaemia
- Sepsis (meningococcal septicaemia needing immediate antibiotics)
- Toxicity, e.g. opiate overdose

Table 5.4 Glasgow Coma Scale and Child's Glasgow Coma Scale

Glasgow Coma Scale (4–15 years)		Child's Glasgow Coma Scale (<4 years)	
Response	Score	Response	Score
Eye opening		*Eye opening*	
Spontaneously	4	Spontaneously	4
To verbal stimuli	3	To verbal stimuli	3
To pain	2	To pain	2
No response to pain	1	No response to pain	1
Best motor response		*Best motor response*	
Obeys verbal command	6	Spontaneous or obeys verbal command	6
Localises to pain	5	Localises to pain or withdraws to touch	5
Withdraws from pain	4	Withdraws from pain	4
Abnormal flexion to pain (decorticate)	3	Abnormal flexion to pain (decorticate)	3
Abnormal extension to pain (decerebrate)	2	Abnormal extension to pain (decerebrate)	2
No response to pain	1	No response to pain	1
Best verbal response		*Best verbal response*	
Orientated and converses	5	Alert; babbles, coos words to usual ability	5
Disorientated and converses	4	Less than usual words, spontaneous irritable cry	4
Inappropriate words	3	Cries only to pain	3
Incomprehensible sounds	2	Moans to pain	2

Management (Figure 5.6)

- Secure the airway
- Give high-flow oxygen
- Support respiration with bag–valve–mask
- Establish intravenous or intraosseous access quickly

TREAT THE TREATABLE. If the history and/or examination suggest opiate overdose is possible, consider treating with naloxone (Figure 5.7). Naloxone has a short half-life, and relapse often occurs after 20 minutes. Further boluses, or an infusion, may be required. Refer to the Appendix for doses.

- Check blood glucose – **DEFG: Don't Ever Forget Glucose**
- Give a broad-spectrum antibiotic, as per local guidelines, to any child in whom sepsis is suspected
- Give a 10 ml/kg rapid bolus of crystalloid to any patient with signs of shock and reassess (5 ml/kg in suspected hyperglycaemia/diabetic ketoacidosis or cardiac causes)
- Undertake appropriate medical management of raised ICP, if noted:
  - nurse with the head in-line in a 30° head-up position (to help cerebral venous drainage)
  - maintain normoglycaemia
  - maintain normal oxygen saturations
  - maintain normothermia when possible
- Transport to definitive care, taking into account the clinical status of the child and avoiding excessive accelerations/decelerations

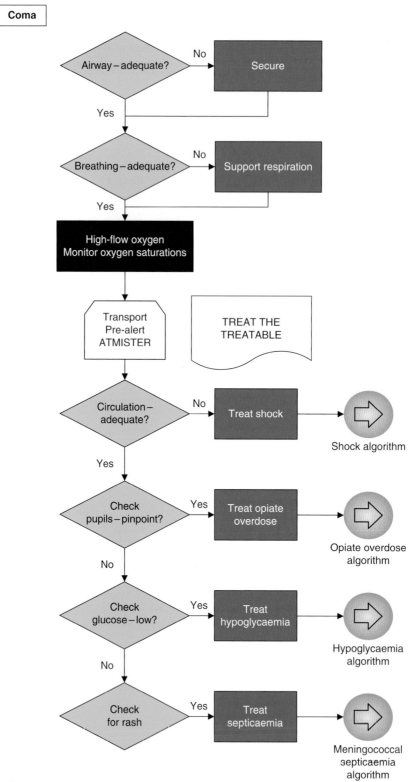

Figure 5.6 Management of coma

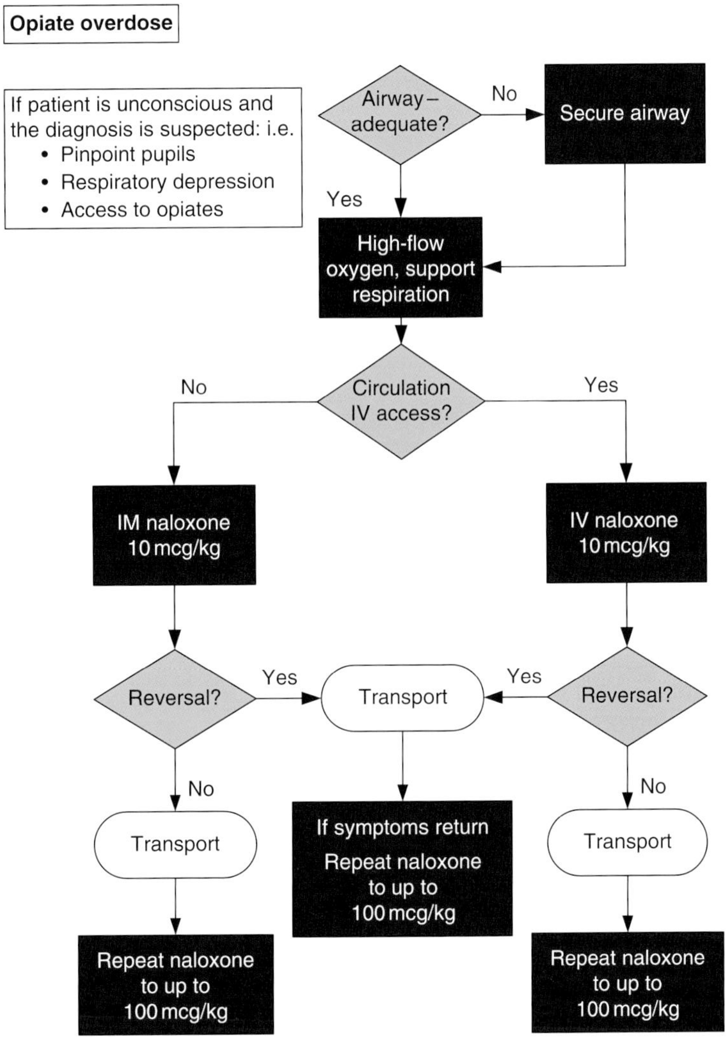

| Opiate overdose |

If patient is unconscious and the diagnosis is suspected: i.e.
- Pinpoint pupils
- Respiratory depression
- Access to opiates

Airway – adequate? — No → **Secure airway**

Yes ↓

High-flow oxygen, support respiration

Circulation IV access?

No → **IM naloxone 10 mcg/kg** → **Reversal?**
- Yes → **Transport** → **If symptoms return Repeat naloxone to up to 100 mcg/kg**
- No → **Transport** → **Repeat naloxone to up to 100 mcg/kg**

Yes → **IV naloxone 10 mcg/kg** → **Reversal?**
- Yes → **Transport**
- No → **Transport** → **Repeat naloxone to up to 100 mcg/kg**

| **Drug doses** |
| Naloxone 10 mcg/kg IV/IM* |
| Subsequent dose up to 100 mcg/kg |
| * Intranasal naloxone can be given at 1 mg per nostril using an atomiser |

Figure 5.7 Management of opiate overdose

Convulsions

Background

Generalised convulsive (tonic–clonic) status epilepticus (CSE) is currently defined as a generalised convulsion lasting 30 minutes or longer or when successive convulsions occur so frequently over a 30-minute period that the patient does not recover consciousness between them. Although the outcome of CSE is mainly determined by its cause, the duration of the convulsion is also relevant. In addition, the longer the duration of the episode, the more difficult it is to terminate it. In general, convulsions that persist beyond 5 minutes may not stop spontaneously, so it is usual practice to institute anticonvulsive treatment when the episode has lasted 5 or more minutes.

Tonic–clonic status occurs in approximately 1–5% of patients with epilepsy. Up to 5% of children with febrile seizures will present with status epilepticus.

Status epilepticus can be fatal, but mortality is lower in children than in adults. Death may be due to complications of the convulsion, such as obstruction of the airway, hypoxia and aspiration of vomit, to overmedication, cardiac arrhythmias or to the underlying disease process.

What to look for

Assess:

- Airway
- Breathing
- Circulation
- Disability – pay particular attention to:
  - mental status/conscious level (AVPU)
  - pupillary size and reaction
  - posture: decorticate or decerebrate posturing in a previously normal child should suggest raised ICP. *These postures can be mistaken for the tonic phase of a convulsion*
- Exposure:
  - rash: if one is present, ascertain if it is purpuric as an indicator of meningococcal disease or non-accidental injury
  - fever: a fever is suggestive evidence of an infectious cause (but its absence does not suggest the opposite) or poisoning with ecstasy, cocaine or salicylates

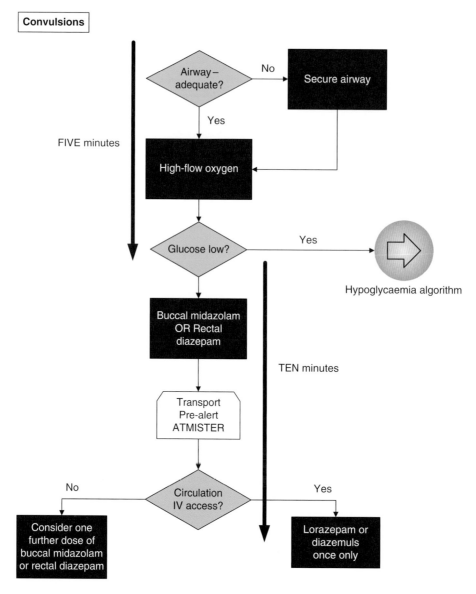

Figure 5.8 Management of convulsions

Management (Figure 5.8)

- Note the time of the convulsion
- Secure the airway
- Give high-flow oxygen
- Check blood glucose and treat hypoglycaemia (2 ml/kg 10% glucose)
- If the convulsion has been going on for at least 5 minutes, give buccal midazolam 0.5 mg/kg or rectal diazepam 0.5 mg/kg
- Gain vascular access, but do not delay transportation to hospital
- One further dose of benzodiazepine may be given 10 minutes after the first dose if needed but must not delay hospital admission
- Be prepared to support ventilation

Hypoglycaemia

Background

Children may become hypoglycaemic because of:

- An excess of insulin or too little carbohydrate as part of the management of diabetes mellitus
- Inadequate stores of glycogen in the face of physiological stress when very ill or injured; the younger the child, the more likely this is to happen
- Sepsis
- Rare metabolic disorders
- Steroid replacement therapy
- Some poisons and drugs (classically alcohol in young children but also β-blockers) can cause hypoglycaemia

What to look for

Any child who is ill enough to need vascular access or has an altered conscious level (especially convulsing) must have a blood glucose measured (hypoglycaemia is present if <3 mmol/l). Some poorly controlled diabetics run chronically high blood sugars and may become symptomatically hypoglycaemic at higher blood sugar levels. Symptoms of hypoglycaemia, as in an adult, may be varied – sweating, pallor, irrational behaviour, aggression, drowsiness, convulsing, etc. all may be seen.

Management (Figure 5.9)

- Take blood for a glucose stick test as above. If in doubt or the test is unavailable, it is safer to treat as if hypoglycaemia is present (<3 mmol/l):
  - if the child is conscious give oral carbohydrates
  - if unable to take oral carbohydrate give a bolus IV of 2 ml/kg 10% glucose. Monitoring glucose levels is mandatory, repeating the bolus if needed
  - glucagon will be relatively ineffective in non-diabetic children

Hyperglycaemia

Background

A high blood sugar is usually due to known or new-onset diabetes mellitus. Sometimes a raised blood sugar is seen after/during severe physiological stress such as a convulsion. This should not be treated. A random sugar of >11 mmol/l is raised.

What to look for

Ask about a history of diabetes. There may have been polyuria (with compensatory polydipsia), weight loss and tiredness. Children nearly always present with type 1 diabetes (insulin dependent) rather than the much more insidious type 2 diabetes. Diabetic ketoacidosis (DKA) occurs when there is a persistent relative lack of insulin for the child's needs. Relatively minor infections sometimes trigger DKA. Once DKA develops, in addition to the symptoms above, the child will have ketones in their urine and breath may smell of pear drops (not everyone can smell this). They will become dehydrated and even shocked from the polyuria, increasingly drowsy and eventually comatose. They may have abdominal pain. The acidosis they develop will lead to respiratory compensation – deep sighing respirations (Kussmaul breathing).

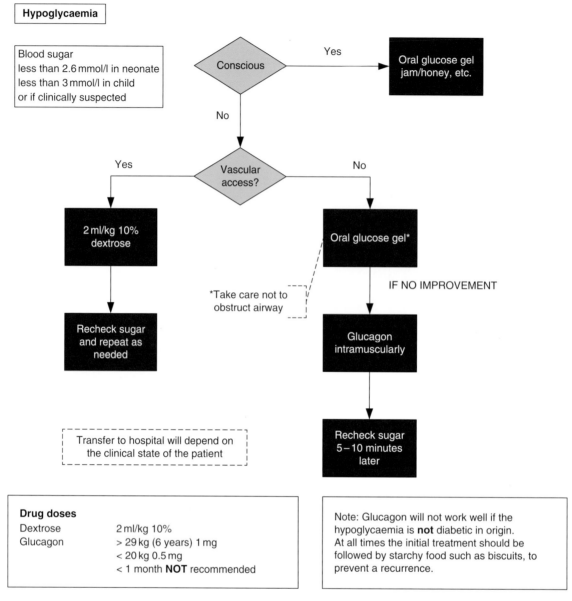

Figure 5.9 Management of hypoglycaemia

Management

Most children with DKA will not need pre-hospital treatment apart from cautious fluid resuscitation in the presence of shock or appropriate management if A, B, C or D is clearly compromised.

Remember: children can die from DKA due to cerebral oedema. Cerebral oedema is unpredictable, occurs more frequently in younger age groups, and about 25% of those affected will die. The cause is not known, but it is believed that a too rapid correction of the dehydration and metabolic abnormalities may contribute.

If the child is very ill, treat according to ABC as follows:

- **Airway** – ensure that the airway is patent and support if required
- If consciousness is reduced, or the child has recurrent vomiting, insert a nasogastric tube, if available and trained, aspirate and leave on open drainage
- **Breathing** – give 100% oxygen by face mask

- **Circulation** – insert an IV cannula and measure sugar level
- Monitor the electrocardiograph
- **Give 5 ml/kg 0.9% (normal) saline as a bolus only if shocked or altered consciousness** (poor peripheral pulses, poor capillary filling with tachycardia and/or hypotension). This can be repeated once if clear signs of shock persist

If the child has severe DKA, do not delay transport and pre-alert the hospital.

Cardiac abnormalities and abnormal rhythms

Background

These are very uncommon in children and most parents/children will be aware of the problem they have and have a protocol as to what to do when they become very ill. Cardiac disease is usually congenital and due to abnormal anatomy; some children will have incomplete oxygenation of their blood – cyanotic congenital heart disease. Their oxygen saturations will always run low and they and their parents will probably know what is right for them. The saturations will not improve significantly with oxygen. Other children have congenital heart disease that does not affect the oxygenation of their blood – they need oxygen if they have low saturations in the normal way but may have equally severe defects.

A few children will have abnormal conducting systems typically leading to recurrent supraventricular tachycardia. Some others will occasionally get ventricular tachycardia or fibrillation – these children may have a prolonged QT interval. Sudden death is a possibility in these children. However, some are now screened as the condition tends to be familial. They may present with recurrent faints or may have been labelled as epileptic. Cardiomyopathy may also lead to arrhythmias and cardiac failure.

What to look for

Listen to the child or parents – this is most reliable!

Cardiac failure is not easy to diagnose outside hospital and very difficult to distinguish from certain causes of respiratory difficulty on occasion. Some of the following signs may be present:

- Signs of shock
- Cyanosis, not correcting with oxygen therapy
- Tachycardia out of proportion to respiratory difficulty
- Raised jugular venous pressure
- Gallop rhythm (3rd heart sound)/murmur
- Enlarged liver
- Absent femoral pulses

A chronic history of breathlessness and tiredness when feeding, along with failure to thrive, should always raise suspicions.

Management (Figures 5.10, 5.11, 5.12, 5.13 and 5.14)

Secure the airway and give high-flow oxygen if needed.

Transport to hospital urgently – pre-alert if the child has respiratory compromise or drowsiness.

If the child has an arrhythmia and is *stable*, pre-hospital treatment is not required other than transport with cardiac monitoring.

Cardiac emergencies

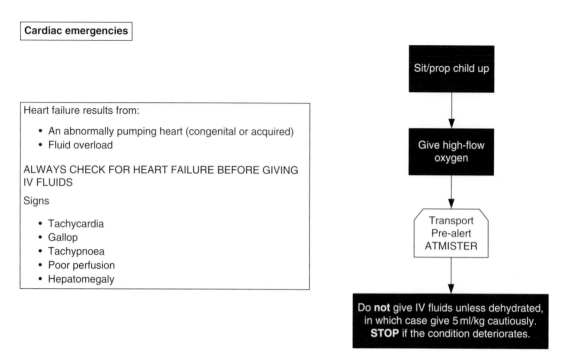

Heart failure results from:

- An abnormally pumping heart (congenital or acquired)
- Fluid overload

ALWAYS CHECK FOR HEART FAILURE BEFORE GIVING IV FLUIDS

Signs

- Tachycardia
- Gallop
- Tachypnoea
- Poor perfusion
- Hepatomegaly

Sit/prop child up

Give high-flow oxygen

Transport Pre-alert ATMISTER

Do **not** give IV fluids unless dehydrated, in which case give 5 ml/kg cautiously. **STOP** if the condition deteriorates.

Figure 5.10 Management of cardiac emergencies

Bradycardia

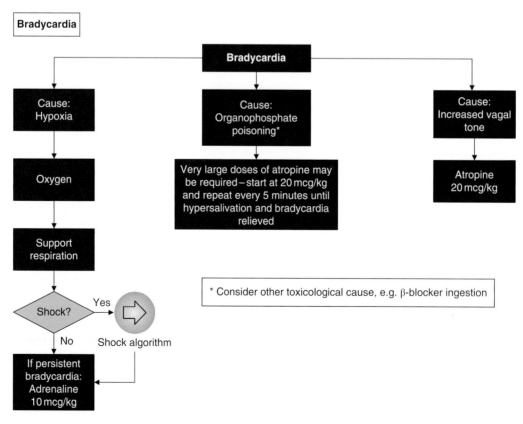

Bradycardia

Cause: Hypoxia

Oxygen

Support respiration

Shock? —Yes→ Shock algorithm

No

If persistent bradycardia: Adrenaline 10 mcg/kg

Cause: Organophosphate poisoning*

Very large doses of atropine may be required – start at 20 mcg/kg and repeat every 5 minutes until hypersalivation and bradycardia relieved

Cause: Increased vagal tone

Atropine 20 mcg/kg

* Consider other toxicological cause, e.g. β-blocker ingestion

Figure 5.11 Management of bradycardia

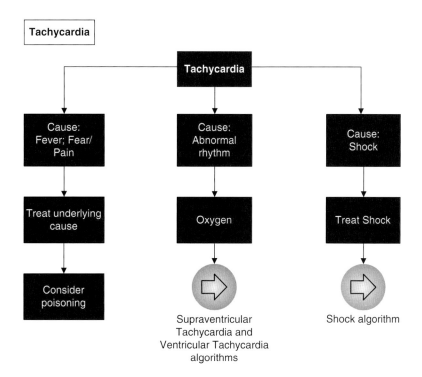

Figure 5.12 Management of tachycardia

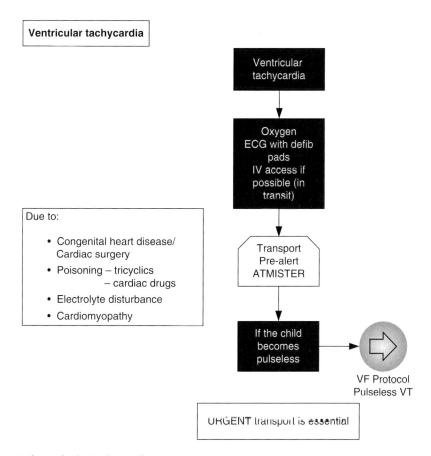

Figure 5.13 Management of ventricular tachycardia

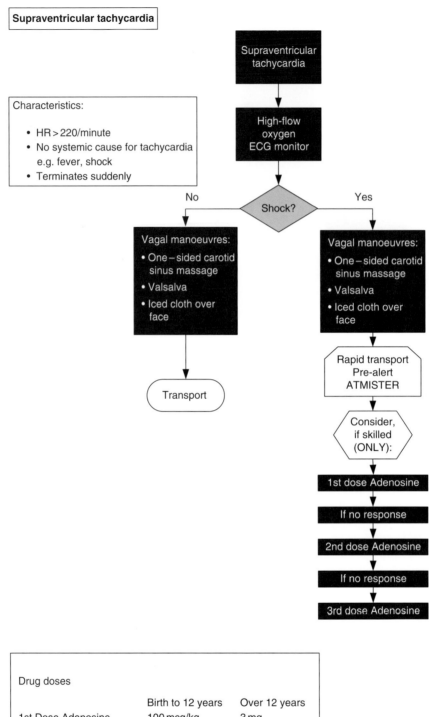

Figure 5.14 Management of supraventricular tachycardia

CHAPTER 6
Structured approach
to the seriously injured child

Learning outcomes

After reading this chapter, you will be able to:
- Describe the pattern of injury in children
- Describe the approach to the resuscitation and emergency treatment of the injured child

---

6.1 Introduction

This chapter sets out a series of algorithms that utilise the structured approach to the initial assessment and management of the seriously injured child, as illustrated in Chapter 4.

As always it is essential that the scene has been assessed and deemed safe before the assessment and management of injuries can begin. Services will vary by location; you should be familiar with your local trauma network.

There is an understandable but probably unnecessarily heightened anxiety associated with providing emergency trauma care to children. Pre-hospital practitioners can be reassured that:

- The structured approach to trauma assessment is the same as in adults: <C> ABCDE
- Experience in adult trauma is transferable to paediatric trauma
- Children get largely the same injuries as adults
- Interventions in paediatric trauma are largely the same as in adult trauma

Pre-hospital trauma scenes are often complex, difficult to control and have a suboptimal environment. This may impair the decisions you make.

By following the principles outlined in the algorithms presented, problems will be identified and treated in order of priority. When dealing with an injured child it is essential that appropriate resuscitative measures are taken as soon as a problem is found. Figure 6.1 and the following box outline the structured approach to pre-hospital patient care.

Systematic approach to pre-hospital patient care

- Primary assessment
- Resuscitation
- Secondary assessment
- Emergency treatment
- Definitive care

Pre-Hospital Paediatric Life Support: A Practical Approach to Emergencies, Third Edition. Edited by Alan Charters, Hal Maxwell and Paul Reavley.
© 2017 John Wiley & Sons Ltd. Published 2017 by John Wiley & Sons Ltd.

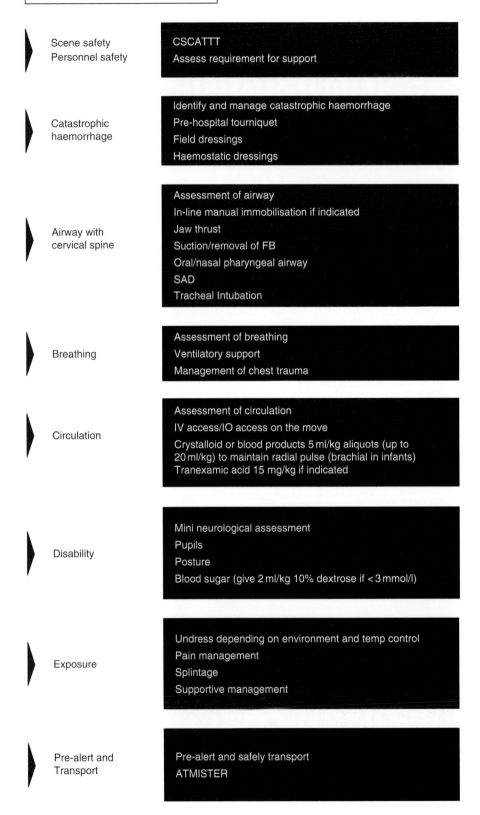

Figure 6.1 **Overall approach to the injured child**

6.2 Assessment

The assessment of the seriously injured child is outlined in Chapter 4 of this manual.

6.3 Treatment

The overall approach is summarised in Figure 6.1 and then detailed in the algorithms for the following presentations:

- Airway injury
- Spinal injury
- Injuries of the pelvis
- Abdominal injury
- Head injury
- Chest injury
- Burns/scalds
- Extremity trauma
- Drowning

Clot preservation

In exsanguinating trauma, the first clot is the strongest clot. Pre-hospital assessment and treatment must be performed in a way to protect any clots already formed or forming.

Minimal handling

- Use scoops and 20° tilts rather than log rolling and sliding
- Avoid unnecessary repeat examinations
- Only move fractures to immobilise them

Good packaging

- Immobilise fractures
- Secure transport of the patient

Measured fluid resuscitation

- 5 ml/kg repeated aliquots
- Repeated reassessment
- Avoid overfilling

Analgesia

Good pain relief is a basic requirement of trauma care. A variety of methods, drugs and routes of administration can be considered. Pharmacological and non-pharmacological methods should be employed (detailed in Chapter 12). The pre-hospital practitioner must have a comprehensive understanding of the drugs and methods available in order to relieve pain.

6.4 Airway injury

Injuries to the airway are very uncommon in children. As the larynx and trachea are soft and pliable, fracture is less likely than in adults so crepitus and obvious disruption may not be detectable in the presence of an injury. Airway injuries obstruct quickly in children so careful assessment is required. Early advanced airway management by a clinician trained in paediatric airway management may be required.

6.5 Spinal injury

Spinal injuries are rare (0.2% of paediatric fractures) but important injuries in children. All severely injured children should be suspected of having a spinal injury. Immobilisation of children is difficult as they are less likely to cooperate with restrictive measures and attempts to implement them may endanger the child further. Spinal immobilisation should be considered in a cooperative child if there is mechanism consistent with injury and:

- Neck pain, or
- Reduced range of movement, or
- Injury above the clavicle, or
- Peripheral neurological deficit

Spinal immobilisation should never interfere with the delivery of immediate life-saving interventions.

Around 80% of spinal injuries in children are cervical, commonly in the upper third. However, the use of cervical spine collars is no longer advocated in children. If immobilisation is assessed as required, then manual in-line stabilisation should be initially provided. If cooperative, blocks and tape should be applied. Immobilisation should not be forced upon the child; fully conscious children are likely to be able to protect their own cervical spine during transfer. Transport should be in either a vacuum mattress or scoop stretcher and never on a spinal board – these are for extraction only. Antiemetics should be considered for all supine and immobilised children (Figure 6.2).

In the very rare occurrence of penetrating cervical injury, immobilisation is not indicated.

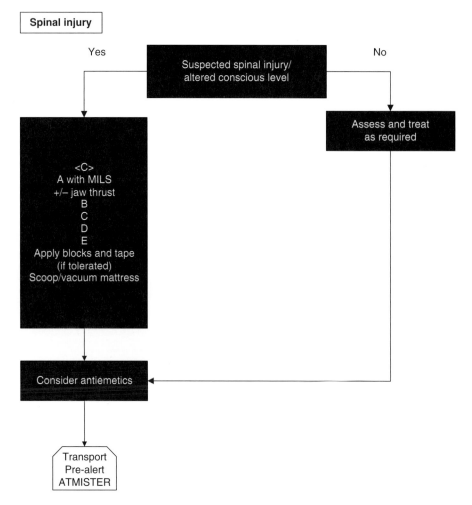

Figure 6.2 Spinal injury treatment algorithm

6.6 Injuries of the pelvis

The incidence of pelvic fractures is around half that seen in adults, but still has a significant mortality of up to 25%. Although the majority of pelvic fractures are stable, the pelvis should be splinted as soon as a fracture is suspected as part of catastrophic haemorrhage management. The principle of clot preservation should be strictly applied.

Pelvic fracture should be suspected when there is:

- High-energy blunt trauma
- Blunt trauma with haemodynamic instability
- Rectal bleeding
- Vaginal bleeding
- Bleeding from the urinary tract
- Pelvic asymmetry
- Pelvic pain
- Pelvic bruising

Pelvic examination should be limited to inspection and very light palpation of the anterior iliac crests to identify asymmetry. There is never any indication for more aggressive manipulation of the pelvic ring to identify fracture. A pelvis should only be examined once.

6.7 Abdominal injury

Blunt trauma causes the majority of abdominal injuries in children. Most occur because of accidents on the roads, while a significant number happen during recreational activities. As always, a detailed pre-hospital history of injury is required to establish the level of likelihood of intra-abdominal injury. A precise history of the mechanism of injury will help in diagnosis. Rapid deceleration, such as experienced during road traffic collisions, causes abdominal compression injuries such as solid organ laceration and deceleration injuries including duodenal tears. Direct blows, such as those caused by punching or an impact with bicycle handlebars, injure the underlying organs. The liver and spleen are less protected and at risk.

There are number of factors that increase the child's susceptibility to intra-abdominal injury.

- Thinner and less muscular abdominal wall offering less protection
- Less thoracic protection
- Less pelvic protection
- Less intraperitoneal fat

An intra-abdominal haemorrhage is non-compressible but in children is less likely to require laparotomy to control bleeding. Preservation of the first clot is vital. In particular care should be taken not to overfill the patient. Transfer to a trauma centre should occur as soon as clinically possible (Figure 6.3).

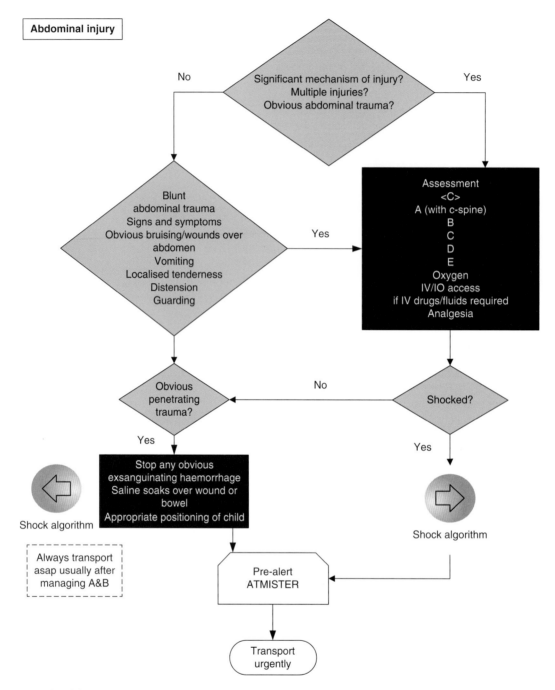

Figure 6.3 Abdominal injury treatment algorithm

6.8 Head injury

The commonest traumatic cause of death in children in the UK is head injury. Road traffic accidents are the commonest mechanism other than in infancy when it is non-accidental injury. Pedestrian children are the most vulnerable, followed by cyclists and then passengers in vehicles. Falls are the second commonest cause of fatal head injuries.

Isolated head trauma should be transferred as per local guidelines. If the patient is stable it is preferable that they are transferred to the nearest paediatric neurosurgical facility, however this may be some distance. If the patient is not stable or not likely to remain stable, they should be taken to the nearest unit with resuscitation and critical care facilities. In the UK patients will be transferred as per the regional trauma network criteria.

Pathophysiology

Brain injury can be divided into primary or secondary. Primary injuries such as haemorrhage, contusion and diffuse axonal injury (DAI) occur at the time of injury and cannot be reversed.

Secondary injury may result from either the secondary effects of cerebral injury or from the cerebral consequences of associated injuries and stress. These may be due to:

- Hypoxia
- Hypercapnia
- Inadequate cerebral perfusion secondary to raised intracranial pressure and/or hypotension
- Hypoglycaemia
- Hypothermia or hyperthermia
- Convulsions

These can be prevented or reduced by early intervention aiming to:

- Maintain adequate ventilation and oxygenation
- Maintain perfusion
- Maintain normoglycaemia

Early critical care support should be considered to provide pre-hospital analgesia. Compression of the neck should be avoided and the patient managed in a 30° head-up position if possible (Figure 6.4).

Raised intracranial pressure

Once the sutures of the skull have closed at 12–18 months of age, the child's cranial cavity behaves like an adult's, with a fixed volume. Cerebral oedema or haematomas increase that volume, but there are initial compensatory mechanisms, e.g. a reduction of the total volume of cerebrospinal fluid (CSF) and the pool of venous blood. When these mechanisms fail, the volume increase leads to a rapid rise in intracranial pressure. This causes an increased pressure gradient for the inflow of arterial blood and a consequent fall in cerebral perfusion pressure:

$$\text{Cerebral perfusion pressure} = \text{Mean systemic BP} - \text{Mean intracranial pressure}$$

As cerebral perfusion falls, further injury secondary to ischaemia results in more oedema. This cycle continues, raising intracranial pressure even further and reducing perfusion. Unchecked this will ultimately result in uncal herniation, coning and death. The clinical signs of this are bradycardia, rising systolic blood pressure with widened pulse pressure and irregular deep respiration. Failure to correct this will result in death. Unilateral increases in intracranial pressure, secondary to haematoma formation, cause ipsilateral uncal herniation. With rising intracranial pressure the third cranial nerve is nipped, causing ipsilateral pupillary dilatation secondary to loss of parasympathetic constrictor tone to the ciliary muscles. This is commonly termed as a 'blown pupil'. If there are any signs of raised intracranial pressure, the administration of hypertonic intravenous fluids can be considered, but should only done with specialist advice. This can be either:

- 20% mannitol solution 1.25–2·5 ml/kg, or
- 3% sodium chloride at 1–2 ml/kg

In childhood, the commonest cause of raised intracranial pressure following head injury is cerebral oedema. Children are especially prone to this problem. They may, of course, also have expanding extradural, subdural or intracerebral haematomas which will require surgical treatment.

Depending on the aetiology of the raised intracranial pressure, definitive treatment is either aimed at preventing secondary injury or removing their causes (surgical intervention).

There are special considerations in infants with head injuries. Their cranial volumes can more easily increase because of unfused sutures. Therefore, large extradural or subdural bleeds may occur before neurological signs or symptoms show; a bulging anterior fontanelle may indicate raised intracranial pressure. Intracranial blood loss in infants can present with signs of hypovolaemia.

If shock is present in the head-injured patient always assume there is an exsanguinating injury elsewhere. This may be from the scalp or elsewhere. The infant's vascular scalp may bleed profusely causing shock.

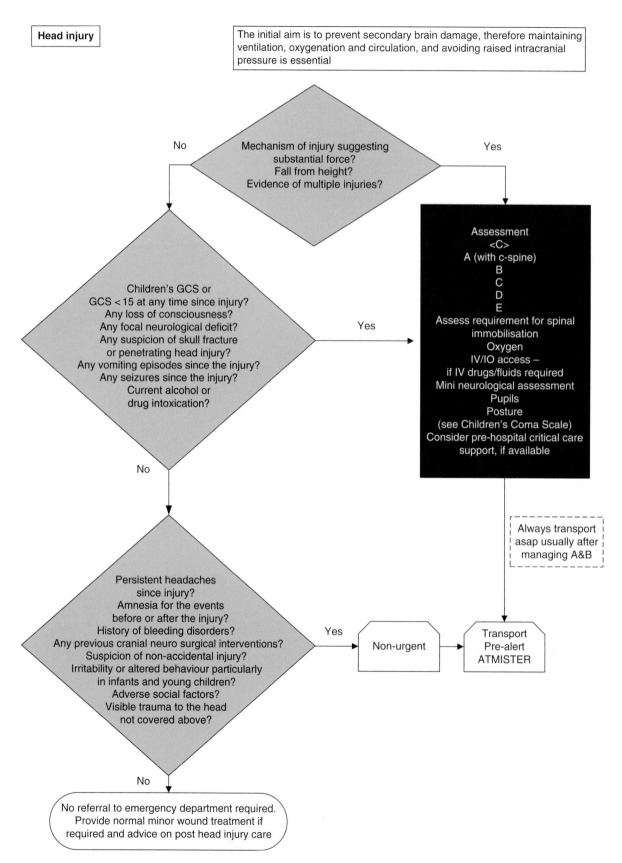

Figure 6.4 Head injury treatment algorithm

The Glasgow and the Children's Coma Scales are shown in Table 6.1.

Table 6.1 Glasgow Coma Scale and Children's Glasgow Coma Scale

Glasgow Coma Scale (4–15 years)		Children's Glasgow Coma Scale (<4 years)	
Response	Score	Response	Score
Eye opening		*Eye opening*	
Spontaneously	4	Spontaneously	4
To verbal stimuli	3	To verbal stimuli	3
To pain	2	To pain	2
No response to pain	1	No response to pain	1
Best motor response		*Best motor response*	
Obeys verbal command	6	Spontaneous or obeys verbal command	6
Localises to pain	5	Localises to pain or withdraws to touch	5
Withdraws from pain	4	Withdraws from pain	4
Abnormal flexion to pain (decorticate)	3	Abnormal flexion to pain (decorticate)	3
Abnormal extension to pain (decerebrate)	2	Abnormal extension to pain (decerebrate)	2
No response to pain	1	No response to pain	1
Best verbal response		*Best verbal response*	
Orientated and converses	5	Alert; babbles, coos words to usual ability	5
Disorientated and converses	4	Less than usual words, spontaneous irritable cry	4
Inappropriate words	3	Cries only to pain	3
Incomprehensible sounds	2	Moans to pain	2

6.9 Chest injury

Following control of catastrophic haemorrhage and airway management, the next consideration in the resuscitation of a child is the assessment of breathing. Chest trauma is the second leading cause of death in children, accounting for between 20% and 30% of major trauma, and thoracic injuries must be considered in all children who suffer major trauma. Some may be life threatening and require immediate therapy during the primary survey and resuscitation, while others may be discovered during the secondary survey. Table 6.2 details the signs associated with different types of chest injury and Figure 6.5 outlines the management procedure.

Most of these children will have other associated injuries. The child who has suffered multiple injuries may well have significant intrathoracic trauma that compromises breathing and requires immediate treatment. The management of traumatic cardiorespiratory arrest in the pre-hospital environment is discussed in Chapter 7.

If the mechanism suggests potential thoracic injury, then it should be very carefully considered. Due to the soft compliant chest wall, substantial amounts of kinetic energy may be transferred through a child's chest wall, resulting in significant intrathoracic injury with little or no external sign of injury.

Because of the mobility of children's organs within the mediastinum, circulatory collapse secondary to tension pneumothorax may develop more quickly than with adults.

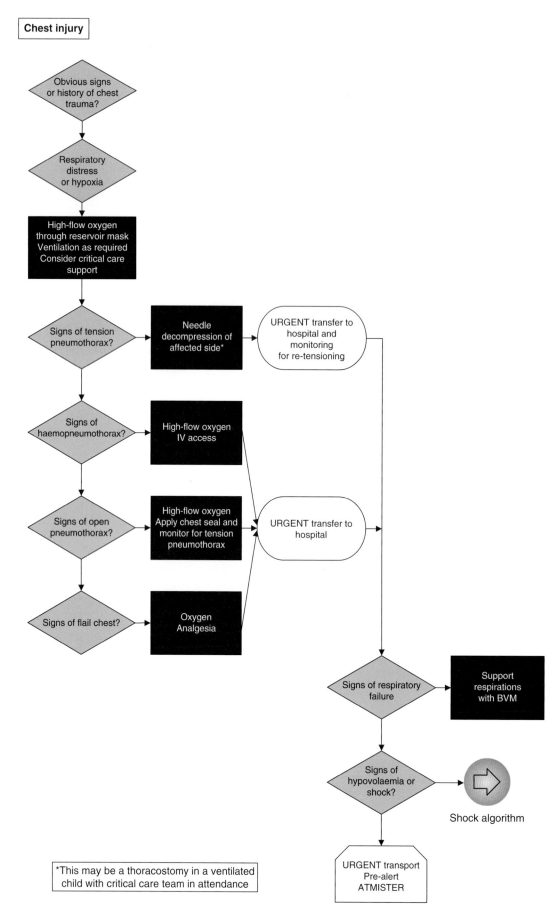

Figure 6.5 Chest injury treatment algorithm

Table 6.2 Signs of chest injuries

Tension pneumothorax	Respiratory distress and hypoxia Shock Decreased air entry/breath sounds on affected side Hyper-resonance to percussion Distended neck veins Tracheal deviation (late sign)
Haemopneumothorax	Respiratory distress Shock Decreased air entry/breath sounds on affected side Decreased chest movement on affected side Dull to percussion on affected side
Open pneumothorax	Penetrating chest wound Respiratory distress and hypoxia Decreased chest movement on affected side Decreased air entry on affected side
Flail chest	Respiratory distress and hypoxia Paradoxical movement of chest wall associated with crepitus
Cardiac tamponade	Severe shock Distended neck veins

6.10 Burns/scalds

Burn injuries are very common in children. Hypovolaemia in the acute setting is very unlikely to be as a result of a burn. It is important to remember that other trauma may accompany burns. Burns are most commonly thermal, but may also be chemical, electrical or radiation in aetiology.

Two main factors determine the severity of thermal burns – the temperature and the duration of contact. The time taken for cellular destruction to occur decreases exponentially with temperature. For example, at 44°C contact would have to be maintained for 6 hours, at 54°C for 30 seconds, and at 70°C epidermal injury happens within a second.

This relationship between temperature and duration of contact underlies the different patterns of injury seen with different types of burn. Scalds generally involve water at below boiling point and contact for less than 4 seconds. Scalds that occur with liquids at a higher temperature (such as hot fat), or in children incapable of minimising the contact time (such as young infants and those with disabilities) tend to result in more serious injuries. Flame burns can involve high temperatures and prolonged contact, and consequently produce the most serious injuries of all. It must be re-emphasised that the most common cause of death, within the first hour following burn injuries, is smoke inhalation. Thus, as with other types of injury, attention to airway and breathing is of prime importance.

First aid is vital for all burns. Thermal burns should be cooled with running tap water as soon as possible for 20 minutes, taking care not to cause hypothermia. Chemical burns should be copiously irrigated, again avoiding hypothermia. Once cooled, the child should have wet clothes or dressings removed and the burns covered with strips of cling film, but not wrapped circumferentially (Figure 6.6).

Burns/scalds

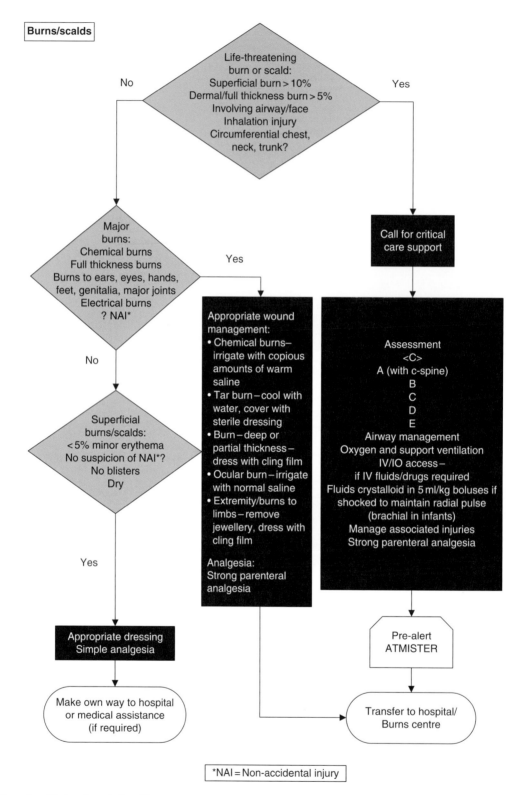

Figure 6.6 Burns/scalds treatment algorithm

The size of burns should be assessed using a paediatric-specific burns chart (Figure 6.7). The percentage area of burns includes partial and deep thickness burns but not superficial or erythematous burns.

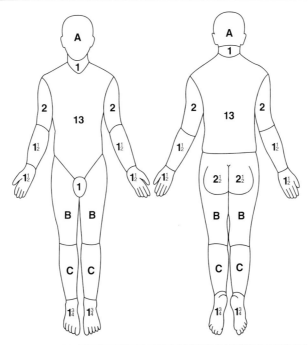

Indicators of inhalation injury

- History of exposure to smoke in a confined space
- Deposits around mouth and nose
- Carbonaceous sputum
- Voice change
- Stridor
- Oral/pharyngeal burns

Immediate and urgent transportation to hospital
Immediate consideration of critical care supports including intubation

Area indicated	Surface area at				
	0	1 year	5 years	10 years	15 years
A	9.5	8.5	6.5	5.5	4.5
B	2.75	3.25	4.0	4.5	4.5
C	2.5	2.5	2.75	3.0	3.25

Figure 6.7 Differences in body surface area (%) in children and indicators of inhalation injury. Source: Artz, 1969. Reproduced with permission of Elsevier

Some paediatric burns will require management in regional centres. Typical criteria for referral to these centres are:

- All burns greater than 1% total body surface area (the size of the child's palm)
- Circumferential burns
- Burns involving the face, hands, perineum or chest
- Burns with inhalational injury including smoke or gas
- Electrical, chemical or radiation burns
- Neonatal burns of any size
- Burns where there are safeguarding concerns

Fluid in burns

If shock is present then fluid resuscitation should commence. Remember that burned patients may also have other injuries causing hypovolaemia.

Burns of more then 15% total body surface area should receive fluids as soon as possible. Mortality is improved with the delivery of fluids within the first hour. If transfer to hospital exceeds 1 hour, fluids should be commenced in the pre-hospital phase. Fluid requirement is calculated using the formula:

$$\text{Percentage burns} \times \text{Weight (kg)} \times 3 = 24\,\text{hour fluid requirement in ml}$$

Half of this volume should be given in the first 8 hours post injury.

Analgesia in burns

Burns are typically very painful and early good analgesia is essential to aid control and assessment. Oral analgesia may not be adequate initially, intravenous access may be difficult and intraosseous access inappropriate unless the child is otherwise unwell. In this circumstance, intranasal diamorphine or intramuscular ketamine (be aware of late absorption in shocked patients) is an excellent route to administer strong pain relief (see Chapter 12).

6.11 Extremity trauma

It is uncommon for extremity trauma to be life threatening in the multiply injured child. It is crucial to recognise and treat associated life-threatening injuries before assessing and managing the skeletal trauma.

The differences between the mature and immature skeleton have a bearing on initial treatment and eventual outcome. Use of the principles usually applied to injuries of the mature skeleton will result in errors of both diagnosis and treatment. Unlike the adult skeleton, which is relatively static, the developing skeleton exhibits structural and functional changes, both physiological and biomechanical, which vary throughout growth. These result in different patterns of fracture, healing response and complications.

It is important to examine both the joint above and below as localising the injury can be difficult due to referred pain or fear of examination. Always start with the opposite, unaffected limb. Give good analgesia as early as possible and consider requirement for radiological imaging. All children who are unable to weight bear following injury require hospital assessment (Figure 6.8).

Unless extremity injury is life threatening, evaluation is carried out during the secondary survey. Single closed extremity injuries may produce enough blood loss to cause hypovolaemic shock but this is not usually life threatening. Multiple fractures can, however, cause severe shock. Closed fractures of the femur may cause loss of approximately 20% of the intravascular volume into the thigh and blood loss from open fractures can be significant. This blood loss begins at the time of the injury and it can be difficult to estimate the degree of pre-hospital loss. Careful assessment at the scene and continuous observation during transportation is therefore necessary.

Traumatic amputation

In the event of a traumatic amputation do the following:

- <C> ABCDE assessment and treatment
- Wrap the amputated part in wet gauze and place in a sterile plastic bag
- Place the bag in crushed ice and water in an insulated container
- Do not allow direct tissue contact with ice
- Transport **with** the patient as soon as clinically safe to do so

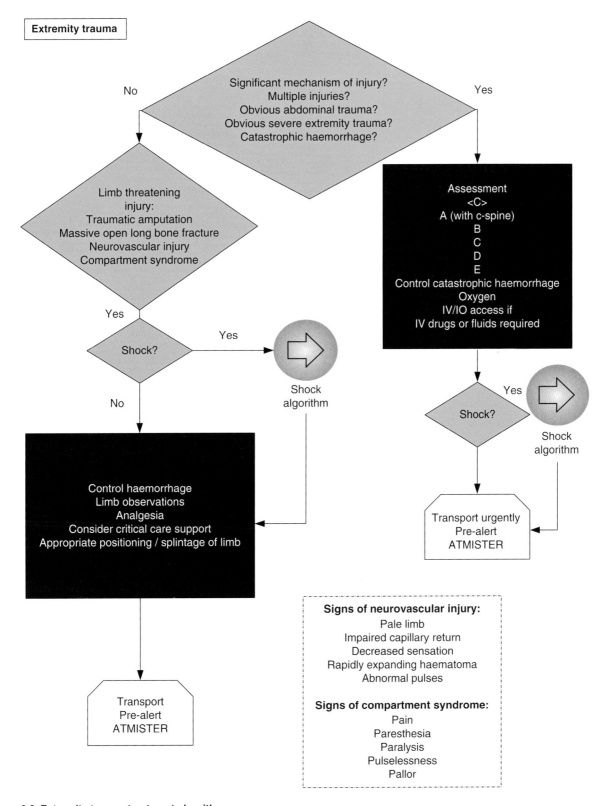

Figure 6.8 Extremity trauma treatment algorithm

Pre-hospital practitioner should be aware of the following paediatric injuries:

Slipped upper femoral epiphysis

This occurs in children approaching or during puberty, between the ages of around 10 and 17 years. It can occur with a relatively low-energy mechanism and may result in necrosis of the femoral head. If it is missed it can have very significant repercussions for the child. It should be excluded by imaging the hip, in any child with a history of trauma, even if minor, who has hip, thigh or knee pain, limping or a restricted range of hip movement.

Toddler's fracture

This occurs in ambulatory children of 9 months to 3 years of age. The mechanism is rotation around a planted foot and it causes a spiral fracture of the tibia. It can result from a very low-energy mechanism and hard clinical signs may be absent. Any previously ambulatory child who suddenly refuses to walk/weight bear should be assessed in hospital.

Supracondylar humeral fracture

Typically seen up to the age of around 10 years and caused by a fall onto the extended arm. This injury is associated with neurovascular injury. Frequently, the injury is obvious with swelling and deformity, but the fracture may be undisplaced. Any child with reduced range of elbow movement following trauma should be transported for hospital assessment.

6.12 Drowning

Drowning is defined as death from asphyxia associated with submersion in a fluid. Near drowning is said to have occurred if there is any recovery (however transient) following a submersion incident.

When a child is first submerged, breath holding occurs and the heart rate slows because of the diving reflex. As apnoea continues hypoxia causes tachycardia, a rise in the blood pressure and acidosis. Between 20 seconds and 2.5 minutes later a break point is reached, and breathing occurs. Fluid is inhaled and on touching the glottis causes immediate laryngeal spasm. Secondary apnoea eventually gives way to involuntary respiratory movements, and water enters the lungs leading to respiratory then cardiac arrest.

Children who survive because of interruption of this chain of events not only require therapy for near drowning, but also assessment and treatment of concomitant hypothermia, electrolyte imbalance and injury (including spinal). Hypothermia is often profound and in the event of the cardiac arrest, the treatment algorithm must be adjusted appropriately (Figure 6.9). If there is severe hypothermia, and if drowning alone and not trauma is the cause of arrest, the patient should be transferred to a unit capable of active re-warming using cardiopulmonary bypass.

Note: If sufficient personnel are available, start the drying and warming process while resuscitation is in progress.

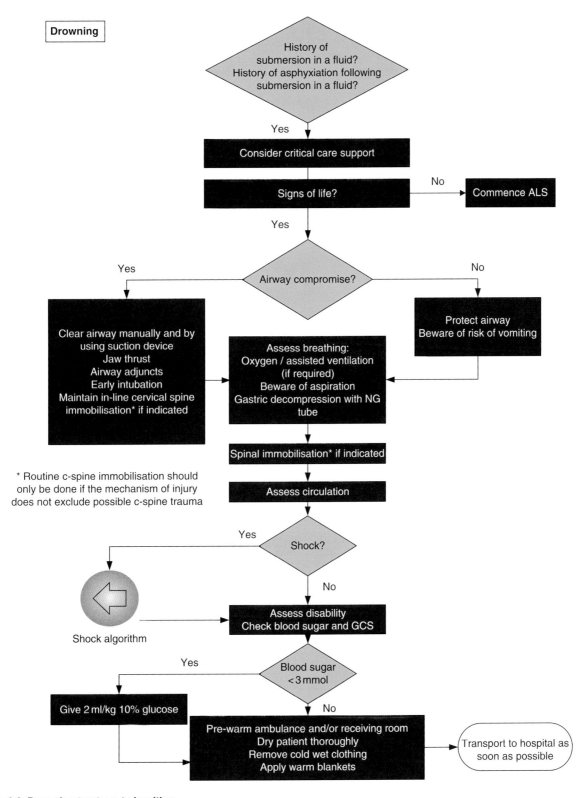

Figure 6.9 Drowning treatment algorithm

6.13 Resuscitation in trauma

A common error in the management of paediatric trauma is to fail to recognise hypovolaemia in children. Careful, structured assessment as previously discussed is required to identify the child that needs fluid resuscitation. Assume that tachypnoea or tachycardia is because of blood loss and not fear, distress or pain in the presence of trauma.

The hospital management of hypovolaemia in trauma now involves the routine use of blood and blood products as the primary resuscitation fluids of choice rather than crystalloids. This is in keeping with the damage control and haemostatic resuscitation strategies thought to improve survival. The aims of resuscitation in trauma are to restore the perfusion of oxygenated blood, prevent coagulopathy, acidosis and hypothermia. Around 15% of paediatric major trauma patients are coagulopathic on arrival at hospital, the presence of which significantly increases mortality. Some pre-hospital critical care systems are now carrying blood and blood products and have the capability to deliver them to the patient already warmed. While blood and blood products will not be routinely available to most trauma victims prior to arrival at hospital, steps can be taken to achieve early availability for the patient. These include early updates to the hospital to trigger the massive transfusion policy and minimising scene time.

In the absence of blood products, pre-hospital practitioners will need to use crystalloids. There is no place for colloids in trauma resuscitation. Use should be carefully considered and measured (see below) as large amounts of crystalloid will cause acidosis, hypothermia and dilution, adding to coagulopathy.

Resuscitation goals

In adult practice, hypotensive resuscitation is well established and improves trauma outcome. A defined period of permissive relative hypotension is observed to allow clot formation and maturation. However, because hypotension occurs late in children and is likely to be due to decompensated shock, we cannot safely use measured hypotension as an end point of resuscitation. Neither is it desirable to attempt to restore normal physiology with large volumes of fluid, particularly crystalloid, in the pre-hospital phase of care. Key points for the first 60 minutes of care post trauma are:

- All fluids in trauma are given in 5 ml/kg aliquots
- The target is a palpable radial pulse (brachial in infants)
- All fluids ideally should be warmed

The early administration of tranexamic acid (TXA) is well established. The Royal College of Paediatrics and Child Health has issued guidance that children with traumatic bleeding should also receive early TXA. Any injured child with suspected blood loss or bleeding and signs of hypovolaemia or actual or predicted requirement for massive transfusion (20 ml/kg) should receive TXA as early as possible. The initial dose of TXA in children is 15 mg/kg IV or IO up to 1 g over 10 minutes.

Traumatic cardiac arrest

This is a rare event but requires a rehearsed and seamless response. The management is discussed in Chapter 7.

CHAPTER 7
Management of cardiac arrest

Learning outcomes

After reading this chapter, you will be able to:
- Demonstrate how to assess the collapsed patient and perform basic life support
- Demonstrate how to manage the choking child
- Demonstrate how to assess the cardiac arrest rhythm and perform advanced life support

---

Although survival rates for children having a cardiac arrest in the pre hospital environment remain poor, immediate and on-going basic life support with effective ventilatory measures have been shown to improve the neurological outcome.

It is essential that effective basic life support is commenced as soon as possible and that the child is transported to an emergency department for on-going support as soon as it is practical to do so.

Basic life support is the foundation on which advanced life support is built. Therefore, it is essential that all advanced life support providers are proficient at basic techniques, and that they are capable of ensuring that basic life support is provided continuously and well during resuscitation.

7.1 Basic life support

Paediatric basic life support (BLS) is not simply a scaled-down version of that provided for adults, although, where possible, guidelines are the same for all ages to aid teaching and retention. Some of the techniques employed need to be varied according to the size of the child. A somewhat artificial line is drawn between infants (less than 1 year old) and children (between 1 year and puberty), and this chapter follows that approach. The preponderance of hypoxic causes of paediatric cardiorespiratory arrest means that oxygen delivery rather than defibrillation is the critical step in children and even in adolescence. This underlines the major differences with the adult algorithm.

By applying the basic techniques described, a single rescuer can support the vital respiratory and circulatory functions of a collapsed child with no equipment. However, health professionals who treat children should use bag–mask ventilation to deliver rescue breaths, if the equipment is provided.

7.2 Primary assessment and resuscitation

Once the child has been approached safely and has been tested for unresponsiveness, assessment and treatment follow the familiar ABC pattern. The overall sequence of BLS in paediatric cardiopulmonary arrest is summarised in Figure 7.1. Note: this guidance is for one or more health professionals. BLS guidance for lay people can be found later in this section.

Pre-Hospital Paediatric Life Support: A Practical Approach to Emergencies, Third Edition. Edited by Alan Charters, Hal Maxwell and Paul Reavley.
© 2017 John Wiley & Sons Ltd. Published 2017 by John Wiley & Sons Ltd.

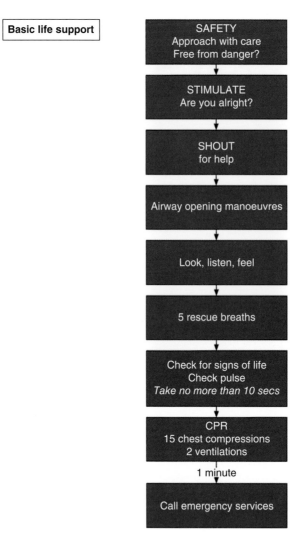

Figure 7.1 Basic life support algorithm

The initial approach: safety, stimulate, shout (SSS)

In the pre-hospital environment, it is essential that the rescuer does not become a second victim, and that the child is removed from continuing danger as quickly as possible. These considerations should precede the initial airway assessment. The steps are summarised in Figure 7.2.

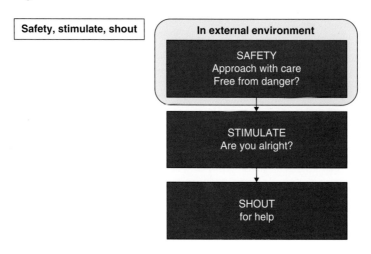

Figure 7.2 Safety, stimulate, shout

Are you alright?

The initial simple assessment of responsiveness consists of asking the child loudly 'Are you alright?' and gently applying a stimulus such as holding the head and shaking the arm. This will avoid exacerbating a possible neck injury whilst still waking a sleeping child. Infants and very small children who cannot talk yet, and older children who are very scared, are unlikely to reply meaningfully, but may make some sound or open their eyes to the rescuer's voice or touch.

Airway (A)

An obstructed airway may be the primary problem, and correction of the obstruction can result in recovery without further intervention. If a child is not breathing it may be because the airway has been blocked by the tongue falling back and obstructing the pharynx. An attempt to open the airway should be made using the head tilt/chin lift manoeuvre. The rescuer places the hand nearest to the child's head on the forehead and applies pressure to tilt the head back gently, whilst the fingers of the other hand are placed on the bony prominence of the chin. The different anatomy of the infant and child makes the desirable degrees of tilt neutral in the infant and sniffing in the child. These are shown in Figures 7.3 and 7.4.

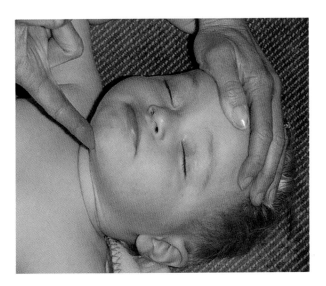

Figure 7.3 Head tilt and chin lift in infants: neutral position

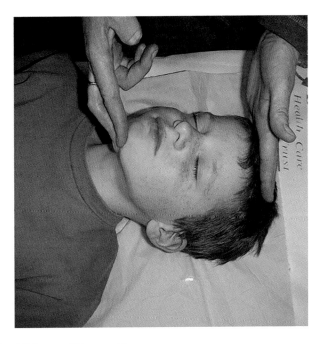

Figure 7.4 Head tilt and chin lift in children: sniffing position

If a child is having difficulty breathing, but is conscious, then transport to hospital should be arranged as quickly as possible. A child will often find the best position to maintain his or her own airway, and should not be forced to adopt a position that may be less comfortable. Attempts to improve a partially maintained airway in a conscious child in an environment where immediate advanced support is not available can be dangerous, because total obstruction may occur.

The patency of the airway should then be assessed. This is done by:

LOOKing	for chest and/or abdominal movement
LISTENing	for breath sounds
FEELing	for breath

It is best achieved by the rescuer placing his or her face above the child's, with the ear over the nose, the cheek over the mouth and the eyes looking along the line of the chest for up to 10 seconds (Figure 7.5).

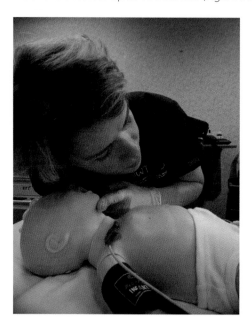

Figure 7.5 Looking, listening, feeling

If the head tilt/chin lift manoeuvre is not possible or is contraindicated because of suspected neck injury, then the jaw thrust manoeuvre can be performed. This is achieved by placing two or three fingers under the angle of the mandible bilaterally and lifting the jaw upwards. This technique may be easier if the rescuer's elbows are resting on the same surface as the child is lying on. A small degree of head tilt may also be applied if there is no concern about neck injury. This is shown in Figure 7.6.

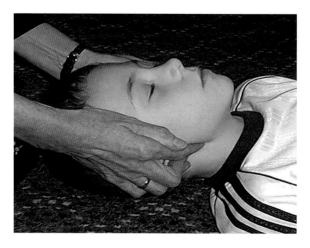

Figure 7.6 Jaw thrust

As before, the success or failure of the intervention is assessed using the technique described above:

- LOOK
- LISTEN
- FEEL

However, on rare occasions, it may not be possible to control the airway with a jaw thrust alone in trauma. In these circumstances, an open airway takes priority over cervical spine risk and a gradually increased degree of head tilt may be tried. Cervical spine control should be achieved by a second rescuer maintaining in-line cervical stabilisation throughout.

The blind finger sweep technique for removal of a foreign body should not be used in children. The child's soft palate is easily damaged, and bleeding from within the mouth can worsen the situation. Furthermore, foreign bodies may be forced further down the airway; they can become lodged below the vocal cords (vocal folds) and be even more difficult to remove. In the child with a tracheostomy, additional procedures are necessary (see Chapter 15).

Breathing (B)

If normal breathing starts after the airway is open, turn the child onto his side in the recovery position (see later in this chapter), maintaining the open airway. Send or go for help and continue to monitor the child for normal breathing. If the airway opening techniques described above do not result in the resumption of adequate breathing within 10 seconds, exhaled air resuscitation should be commenced. The rescuer should distinguish between adequate breathing and ineffective, gasping or obstructed breathing. If in doubt, attempt rescue breathing.

Five initial rescue breaths should be given

While the airway is kept open as described, the rescuer breathes in and seals his or her mouth around the victim's mouth (for a child), or mouth and nose (for an infant, as shown in Figure 7.7). If the mouth alone is used then the nose should be pinched closed using the thumb and index fingers of the hand that is maintaining the head tilt. Slow exhalation (1 second) by the rescuer should make the victim's chest visibly rise – too vigorous a breath will cause gastric insufflation and increase the chance of regurgitation of stomach contents into the lungs and may also cause gastric splinting of the diaphragm, which will impede good ventilation. The rescuer should take a breath between rescue breaths to maximise oxygenation of the victim.

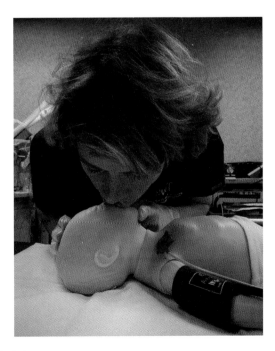

Figure 7.7 Mouth to mouth and nose in infants

If the rescuer is unable to cover the mouth and nose in an infant, he or she may attempt to seal only the infant's nose or mouth with his or her mouth and should close the infant's lips or pinch the nose to prevent air escape.

General guidance for exhaled air resuscitation

- The chest should be seen to rise
- Inflation pressure may be higher because the airway is small
- Slow breaths at the lowest pressure reduce gastric distension
- As soon as possible change to a self-inflating bag

If the chest does not rise, then the airway is not clear. The usual cause is failure to apply correctly the airway opening techniques discussed. Thus, the first thing to do is to readjust the head tilt/chin lift position, and try again. If this does not work, a jaw thrust should be tried. It is quite possible for a single rescuer to open the airway using this technique and perform exhaled air resuscitation. Five rescue breaths are given. While performing rescue breaths, note any gag or cough response to your action. These responses, or their absence, will form part of your assessment of 'signs of life' described below.

Failure of both the head tilt/chin lift and jaw thrust should lead to the suspicion that a foreign body is causing the obstruction, and appropriate action should be taken (see Section 7.4).

Circulation (C)

Once the rescue breaths have been given, attention should be turned to the circulation.

Assessment

Failure of the circulation is recognised by the absence of signs of circulation ('signs of life'), i.e. no normal breaths or cough in response to rescue breaths and no spontaneous movement. In addition, the absence of a central pulse for up to 10 seconds or the presence of a pulse at an insufficient rate (less than 60 with no signs of circulation) may be detected.

The absence of 'signs of life' is the primary indication to start chest compressions. Signs of life include: movement, coughing or normal breathing (not agonal gasps – these are irregular, infrequent breaths). Experienced health professionals can find it difficult to be certain that the pulse is absent within 10 seconds, therefore, unless you are certain you feel a pulse, start chest compressions.

In children the carotid artery in the neck or the femoral artery in the groin can be palpated. In infants the neck is generally short and fat and the carotid artery may be difficult to identify. Therefore the brachial artery in the medial aspect of the antecubital fossa, or the femoral artery in the groin, can be felt.

Start chest compressions if within 10 seconds:

- There are no signs of life
- You are not certain if there is a pulse
- There is a slow pulse (less than 60 beats per minute with no signs of circulation and no reaction to ventilation)

In the absence of signs of life, chest compressions must be started unless you are certain that you can feel a pulse of more than 60 beats per minute within 10 seconds. 'Unnecessary' chest compressions are almost never damaging and it is important not to waste vital seconds before starting them. If the pulse is present – and has an adequate rate, with good perfusion – but apnoea persists, exhaled air resuscitation must be continued until spontaneous breathing resumes.

Chest compressions

For the best effect the child must be placed lying flat on his or her back, on a firm surface. Children vary in size, and the exact nature of the compressions given should reflect this. In general, infants (less than 1 year old) require a technique different from children up to puberty in whom the method used in adults can be applied with appropriate modifications for their size. Compressions should be at least one-third of the depth of the child's (5 cm) or infant's (4 cm) chest.

Position for chest compressions

Chest compressions should compress the lower half of the sternum, but avoid placing the hand/fingers too low, thus pressing the xiphisternum in the abdomen. Of equal importance is to ensure that the chest wall fully recoils before the next compression starts – this will ensure that coronary arteries fill.

Infants

Infant chest compression can be more effectively achieved using the hand-encircling technique: the infant is held with both the rescuer's hands encircling or partially encircling the chest. The thumbs are placed over the lower half of the sternum and compression is carried out, as shown in Figure 7.8. This method is only possible when there are two rescuers, as the time needed to reposition the airway precludes its use by a single rescuer if the recommended rates of compression and ventilation are to be achieved. The single rescuer should use the two-finger method, placing two fingers on the lower half of the sternum and employing the other hand to maintain the airway position as shown in Figure 7.9.

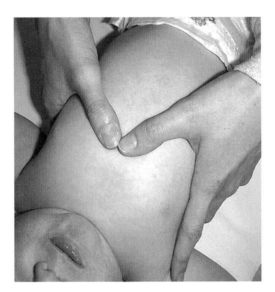

Figure 7.8 Hand-encircling technique

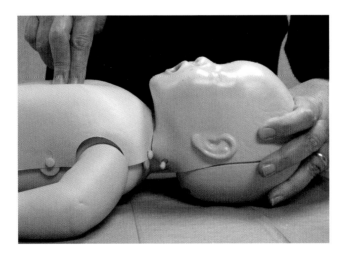

Figure 7.9 Chest compressions in an infant

Children

Place the heel of one hand over the lower half of the sternum. Lift the fingers to ensure that pressure is not applied over the child's ribs. Position yourself vertically above the child's chest and, with your arm straight, compress the sternum to depress it by at least one-third of the depth of the chest or by 5 cm (Figure 7.10). For larger children, or for small rescuers, this may be achieved most easily by using both hands with the fingers interlocked (Figure 7.11). The rescuer may choose one or two hands to achieve the desired compression of at least one-third of the depth of the chest.

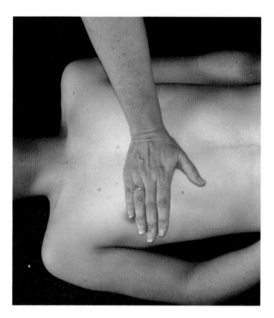

Figure 7.10 Chest compressions: one handed

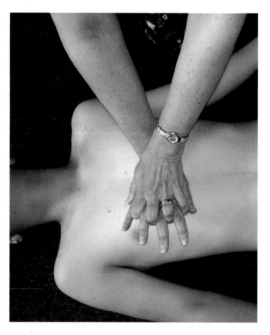

Figure 7.11 Chest compressions: two handed

Once the correct technique has been chosen and the area for compression identified, 15 compressions should be given to two ventilations.

Compression : ventilation ratios

Experimental work has shown that coronary perfusion pressure in resuscitation increases if sequences of compressions are prolonged rather than curtailed. Equally, ventilations are a vital part of all resuscitation procedures and are needed early, especially in the hypoxic/ischaemic arrests characteristic of childhood. Once BLS has started, interruptions to chest compressions should only be for ventilations. Pausing compressions will decrease coronary perfusion pressure to zero and several compressions will be required before adequate coronary perfusion recurs. There is no experimental evidence to support any particular ratio in childhood but a 15:2 ratio has been validated by experimental and mathematical studies and is the recommended ratio for healthcare professionals.

Where possible, once the child has either been intubated or a SAD with an effective seal is placed during advanced life support, asynchronous compressions may be carried out with a ventilation rate of 10–12 breaths per minute.

Continuing cardiopulmonary resuscitation

The compression rate at all ages is 100–120 per minute. A ratio of 15 compressions to two ventilations is maintained whatever the number of rescuers. If possible, change rescuers every 2 minutes to maintain optimal compressions. If no help has arrived the emergency services must be contacted after 1 minute of cardiopulmonary resuscitation (CPR). With pauses for ventilation there will be less than 100–120 compressions per minute although the **rate** is 100–120 per minute. Compressions can be recommended at the end of inspiration and may augment exhalation. Apart from this interruption to summon help, BLS must not be interrupted unless the child moves or takes a breath.

Research on the delivery of CPR has shown that rescuers tend to compress too slowly and too gently. So the current emphasis is on CPR that is 'hard and fast' with compressions of at least one-third of the victim's anteroposterior chest diameter and a rate of between 100 and 120 compressions a minute, minimising interruptions as completely as possible. Any time spent readjusting the airway or re-establishing the correct position for compressions will seriously decrease the number of cycles given per minute. This can be a very real problem for the solo rescuer, and there is no easy solution. In the infant and small child, the free hand can maintain the head position. The correct position for compressions does not need to be re-measured after each ventilation.

In the older child, biometric devices may be used which give feedback on the quality and speed of chest compressions – unless the application of such devices causes a delay in compressions.

The CPR manoeuvres recommended for infants and children are summarised in Table 7.1.

Table 7.1 Summary of basic life support techniques in infants and children

	Infant (<1 year)	Child (1 year to puberty)
Airway		
Head-tilt position	Neutral	Sniffing
Breathing		
Initial slow breaths	Five	Five
Circulation		
Pulse check	Brachial or femoral	Carotid or femoral
Landmark	Lower half of sternum	Lower half of sternum
Technique	Two fingers or two thumbs	One or two hands
CPR ratio	15:2	15:2

Age definitions

As the techniques of CPR have been simplified there is now no need to distinguish between different ages of children but only between infants (under 1 year) and children (from 1 year to puberty). It is clearly inappropriate and also unnecessary to establish the physical evidence for puberty at CPR. The rescuer should use paediatric guidelines if he or she believes the victim to be a child. If the victim is, in fact, a young adult, no harm will be caused as the aetiology of cardiac arrest is, in general, similar in this age group to that in childhood, i.e. hypoxic/ischaemic rather than cardiac in origin.

Recovery position

No specific recovery position has been identified for children. An example of one recovery position is shown in Figure 7.12. The child should be placed in a stable, lateral position that ensures maintenance of an open airway with free drainage of fluid from the mouth, the ability to monitor and gain access to the patient, security of the cervical spine and attention to pressure points.

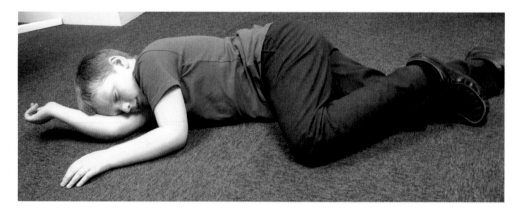

Figure 7.12 Example recovery position

The following is a description of the technique for adults and is suitable for children:

- Kneel beside the victim and make sure that both his legs are straight
- Place the arm nearest to you out at right angles to his body, elbow bent with the hand palm up
- Bring the far arm across the chest, and hold the back of the hand against the victim's cheek nearest to you
- With your other hand, grasp the far leg just above the knee and pull it up, keeping the foot on the ground
- Keeping his hand pressed against his cheek, pull on the far leg to roll the victim towards you on to his side
- Adjust the upper leg so that both the hip and knee are bent at right angles
- Tilt the head back to make sure that the airway remains open
- If necessary, adjust the hand under the cheek to keep the head tilted and facing downwards to allow liquid material to drain from the mouth
- Check breathing regularly
- If the victim has to be kept in the recovery position for more than 30 minutes turn him to the opposite side to relieve the pressure on the lower arm

Lay rescuers

Bystander CPR is associated with better neurological outcome in adults and children than no CPR intervention. However, it has become clear that bystanders often do not undertake BLS because they are afraid to do it wrongly and because of an anxiety about performing mouth-to-mouth resuscitation on strangers. For lay rescuers, therefore, the adult compression : ventilation ratio of 30 compressions to two ventilations is recommended for children as well as adults, thus simplifying the guidance. To increase the appropriateness for children, lay rescuers should be advised to precede their efforts by five rescue breaths if the victim is a child. If lay rescuers are unable or unwilling to perform mouth-to-mouth resuscitation, they may perform compression-only CPR. Single healthcare professional rescuers are also encouraged to perform five rescue breaths followed by a ratio of 30 compressions to two ventilations for children if they find difficulty in the transition from compressions to ventilations.

Automatic external defibrillators in children

The use of the automatic external defibrillator (AED) is now included in BLS teaching for adults because early defibrillation is the most effective intervention for the large majority of unpredicted cardiac arrests in adults. As has been stated, in children and young people, circulatory or respiratory causes of cardiac arrest predominate. However, in certain circumstances, children may suffer a primary cardiac cause for cardiac arrest, and the use of an AED may be life saving. Recently, there has been a large increase in the number of AEDs, together with trained operators, made available in public places such as airports, places of entertainment and shops, so the opportunity for their use will correspondingly increase.

7.3 Basic life support and infection risk

There have been a few reports of the transmission of infectious diseases from casualties to rescuers during mouth-to-mouth resuscitation. The most serious concern in children is meningococcus, and rescuers involved in the resuscitation of the airway in such patients should take standard prophylactic antibiotics (rifampicin or ciprofloxacin). Tuberculosis can be transmitted during CPR and appropriate precautions should be taken when this is suspected.

There have been no reported cases of transmission of human immunodeficiency virus (HIV) through mouth-to-mouth ventilation. Blood-to-blood contact is the single most important route of transmission of such viruses, and in non-trauma resuscitations the risks are negligible. Sputum, saliva, sweat, tears, urine and vomit are low-risk fluids. Precautions should be taken, if possible, in cases where there might be contact with blood, semen, vaginal secretions, cerebrospinal fluid, pleural and peritoneal fluids and amniotic fluid. Precautions are also recommended if any bodily secretion contains visible blood. Devices that prevent direct contact between the rescuer and the victim (such as resuscitation masks) can be used to lower risk; gauze swabs or any other porous material placed over the victim's mouth is of no benefit in this regard.

The number of children in the UK with acquired immune deficiency syndrome (AIDS) or HIV-1 infection is less than the number of adults similarly affected. If transmission of HIV-1 does occur in the UK, it is therefore much more likely to be from the adult rescuer to the child rather than the other way around.

In countries where HIV/AIDS is more prevalent, the risk to the rescuer will be greater. In South Africa, in a medical ward 25–40% of children may be HIV-positive but the prevalence is lower in trauma cases. In the Caribbean, HIV prevalence is second only to sub-Saharan Africa. The situation may change as effective antiretroviral agents are made available to resource-poor countries.

7.4 The choking child

The vast majority of deaths from foreign body airway obstruction (FBAO) occur in pre-school children. Virtually anything may be inhaled, foodstuffs predominating. The diagnosis may not be clear-cut, but should be suspected if the onset of respiratory compromise is sudden and is associated with coughing, gagging and stridor.

Airway obstruction also occurs with infections such as acute epiglottitis and croup. In these cases, attempts to relieve the obstruction using the methods described below are dangerous. Children with known or suspected infectious causes of obstruction, and those who are still breathing and in whom the cause of obstruction is unclear, should be taken to hospital urgently. The treatment of these children is dealt with in Chapter 5.

If a foreign body is easily visible and accessible in the mouth then remove it, but while attempting this take great care not to push it further into the airway. Do not perform blind finger sweeps of the mouth or upper airway as these may further impact a foreign body and damage tissues without removing the object.

The physical methods of clearing the airway described here should therefore only be performed if:

1. The diagnosis of FBAO is clear-cut (witnessed or strongly suspected) and ineffective coughing and increasing dyspnoea, loss of consciousness or apnoea have occurred
2. Head tilt/chin lift and jaw thrust have failed to open the airway of an apnoeic child. (The sequence of instructions is shown in Figure 7.13)

If the child is coughing he should be encouraged. A spontaneous cough is more effective at relieving an obstruction than any externally imposed manoeuvre. An effective cough is recognised by the victim's ability to speak or cry and to take a breath between coughs. The child should be continually assessed and not left alone at this stage. No intervention should be made unless the cough becomes ineffective, that is quieter or silent, and the victim cannot cry, speak or take a breath or if he becomes cyanosed or starts to lose consciousness. Then call for help and start the intervention.

These manoeuvres are then alternated with each other and with examination of the mouth and attempted breaths, as shown in Figure 7.13.

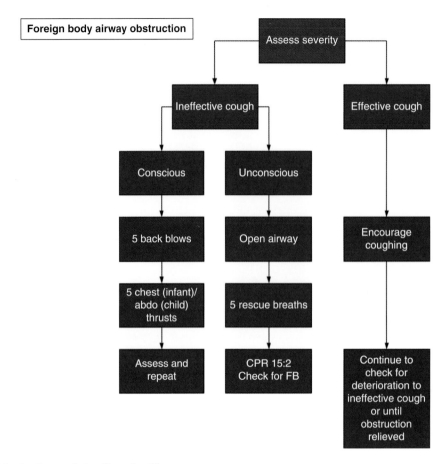

Figure 7.13 Foreign body airway obstruction algorithm

Infants

Abdominal thrusts may cause intra-abdominal injury in infants. Therefore, a combination of back blows and chest thrusts is recommended for the relief of FBAO in this age group.

The baby is placed along one of the rescuer's arms in a head-down position, with the rescuer's hand supporting the infant's jaw in such a way as to keep it open, in the neutral position. The rescuer then rests his or her arm along the thigh, and delivers five back blows between the shoulder blades with the heel of the free hand.

If the obstruction is not relieved the baby is turned over and laid along the rescuer's thigh, still in a head-down position. Five chest thrusts are given – using the same landmarks as for cardiac compression but at a slower rate of one per second and sharper than chest compressions. If an infant is too large to allow use of the single-arm technique described above, then the same manoeuvres can be performed by laying the baby across the rescuer's lap. These techniques are shown in Figures 7.14 and 7.15.

Children

Back blows can be used as in infants or, in the case of a larger child, with the child supported in a forward leaning position (Figure 7.16).

In the child the abdominal thrust (Heimlich manoeuvre) can also be used. This can be performed with the victim either standing or lying, but the former is usually more appropriate. If this is to be attempted with the child standing, the rescuer moves behind the victim and passes his or her arms around the victim's body. Owing to the short height of children, it may be necessary for an adult to raise the child or kneel behind them to carry out the standing manoeuvre effectively. One hand is formed into a fist and placed against the child's abdomen above the umbilicus and below the xiphisternum. The other hand is placed over the fist, and both hands are thrust sharply upwards into the abdomen. This is repeated five times unless the object causing the obstruction is expelled before then.

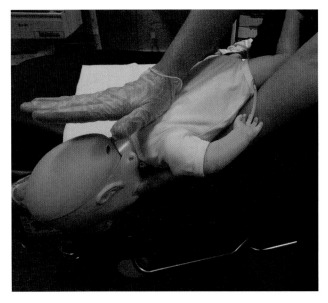

Figure 7.14 Back blows

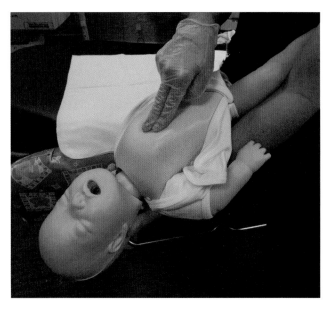

Figure 7.15 Chest thrusts

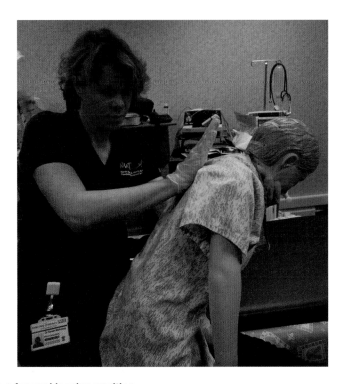

Figure 7.16 Child supported in a forward leaning position

To carry out the Heimlich manoeuvre in a supine child, the rescuer kneels at his or her feet. If the child is large it may be necessary to kneel astride him or her. The heel of one hand is placed against the child's abdomen above the umbilicus and below the xiphisternum. The other hand is placed on top of the first, and both hands are thrust sharply upwards into the abdomen, with care being taken to direct the thrust in the midline. This is repeated five times unless the object causing the obstruction is expelled before that. This technique is shown in Figure 7.17.

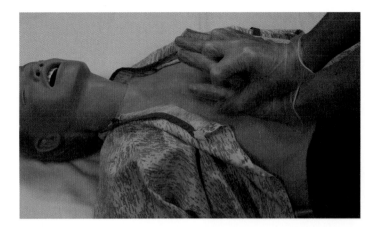

Figure 7.17 Heimlich manoeuvre in a supine child

Following successful relief of the obstructed airway, assess the child clinically. There may be still some part of the foreign material in the respiratory tract. If abdominal thrusts have been performed, the child should be assessed for possible abdominal injuries.

Each time breaths are attempted, look in the mouth for the foreign body and remove it if visible. Take care not to push the object further down and avoid damaging the tissues. If the obstruction is relieved, the victim may still require either continued ventilations if not breathing but is moving or gagging or both ventilations and chest compressions if there are no signs of life. Advanced life support may also be needed.

If the child breathes effectively then place in the recovery position and continue to monitor regularly.

In the unconscious infant or child with FBAO:

- Call for help
- Place the child supine on a flat surface
- Open the mouth and attempt to remove any visible object
- Open the airway and attempt five rescue breaths, repositioning the airway with each breath if the chest does not rise
- Start chest compressions even if the rescue breaths were ineffective
- Continue the sequence for single-rescuer CPR for about a minute then summon help again if none is forthcoming

7.5 Advanced life support

Cardiac arrest has occurred when there is no effective cardiac output. Before any specific therapy is started, effective BLS must be established. The priority for the pre-hospital provider is to establish effective BLS and transfer the child to hospital as soon as practically possible.

Four cardiac arrest rhythms will be discussed in this chapter:

1. Asystole
2. Pulseless electrical activity (also known as electromechanical dissociation)
3. Ventricular fibrillation
4. Pulseless ventricular tachycardia

The four are divided into two groups: two that do not require defibrillation (called 'non-shockable') and two that do require defibrillation ('shockable') (Figure 7.18).

```
                           ┌──────────────────────────┐
  ┌──────────────┐         │          SAFETY          │
  │ Cardiac arrest │        │     Approach with care    │
  └──────────────┘         │      Free from danger?    │
                           └──────────────────────────┘
                                        │
                           ┌──────────────────────────┐
                           │        STIMULATE          │
                           │     Are you alright?      │
                           └──────────────────────────┘
                                        │
                           ┌──────────────────────────┐
                           │          SHOUT            │
                           │         for help          │
                           └──────────────────────────┘
                                        │
                           ┌──────────────────────────┐
                           │     Airway opening        │
                           │       manoeuvres          │
                           └──────────────────────────┘
                                        │
                           ┌──────────────────────────┐
                           │     Look, listen, feel    │
                           └──────────────────────────┘
                                        │
                           ┌──────────────────────────┐
                           │      5 rescue breaths     │
                           └──────────────────────────┘
                                        │
                    ┌────────────────────────────────────┐
                    │     Check for signs of life         │
                    │          Check pulse                │
                    │    Take no more than 10 secs        │
                    └────────────────────────────────────┘
                                        │
                    ┌────────────────────────────────────┐
                    │               CPR                   │
                    │  15 chest compressions : 2 ventilations │
                    └────────────────────────────────────┘
                                        │
            VF/                         ◆                  Asystole/
        pulseless VT               Assess rhythm             PEA
  ┌──────────────┐    ◀──────────    ◆    ──────────▶  ┌──────────────┐
  │  Shockable   │                                      │ Non-shockable │
  └──────────────┘                                      └──────────────┘
```

Figure 7.18 Cardiac arrest algorithm

7.6 Non-shockable rhythms

This includes asystole and pulseless electrical activity.

Asystole

This is the most common arrest rhythm in children, because the response of the young heart to prolonged severe hypoxia and acidosis is progressive bradycardia leading to asystole (Figure 7.19). The electrocardiogram (ECG) will distinguish asystole from ventricular fibrillation, ventricular tachycardia and pulseless electrical activity (PEA). The ECG appearance of ventricular asystole is an almost straight line; occasionally P-waves are seen. Check that the appearance is not caused by an artefact (e.g. a loose wire or disconnected electrode); however modern defibrillators will indicate disconnection with a broken rather than continuous line. Turn up the gain on the ECG monitor.

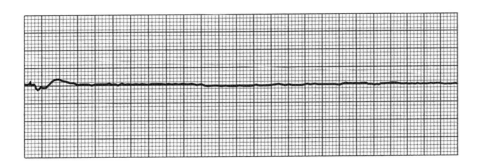

Figure 7.19 Asystole

Pulseless electrical activity

This is the absence of signs of life or a palpable pulse despite the presence on the ECG monitor of recognisable complexes that normally produce perfusion (Figure 7.20). PEA is treated in the same way as asystole and is often a pre-asystolic state.

Pulseless electrical activity may be due to an identifiable and reversible cause. In children, the most common causes are hypovolemia and hypoxia. Trauma is also most often associated with a reversible cause of PEA. This may be due to severe hypovolaemia, tension pneumothorax or pericardial tamponade. PEA is also seen in hypothermic patients and in patients with electrolyte abnormalities, including hypocalcaemia from calcium channel blocker overdose. Rarely in children, it may be seen after massive pulmonary thromboembolus.

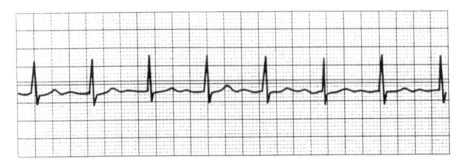

Figure 7.20 Pulseless electrical activity

Management of asystole/PEA

The first essential is to establish ventilations and chest compressions effectively. Ventilations are provided initially by bag-and-mask with high-concentration oxygen. Ensure a patent airway, initially using an airway manoeuvre to open the airway and stabilising it with an airway adjunct.

Provide effective chest compressions at a rate of 100–120 per minute with a compression : ventilation ratio of 15:2. The depth of compression should be at least one-third of the anteroposterior diameter of the chest (4 cm for infants, 5 cm for children). The child should have a cardiac monitor attached and the heart's rhythm assessed.

Although the procedures to stabilise the airway and gain circulatory access are now described sequentially, they should be undertaken simultaneously under the direction of a resuscitation team leader. The role of the team leader is to coordinate care and to anticipate problems in the sequence.

If asystole or PEA is identified give adrenaline 10 micrograms/kg IV or IO. Adrenaline is the first-line drug for asystole. Through α-adrenergic-mediated vasoconstriction, its action is to increase aortic diastolic pressure during chest compressions and thus coronary perfusion pressure and the delivery of oxygenated blood to the heart. It also enhances the contractile state of the heart and stimulates spontaneous contractions. The intravenous or intraosseous dose is 10 micrograms/kg (0.1 ml/kg of 1:10 000 solution). Whenever venous access is not attainable within 1 minute, intraosseous access should be used. Central lines provide more secure long-term access, but compared to intraosseous or peripheral intravenous access offer no advantages. In each case the adrenaline is followed by a normal saline flush (2–5 ml).

If circulatory access cannot be gained, the tracheal tube is a last resort option, but the absorption is highly variable and it should be avoided if possible. If used, the drug should be injected quickly down a narrow-bore suction catheter in 10 times the intravenous dose beyond the tracheal end of the tube and then flushed in with 1 or 2 ml of normal saline.

As soon as is feasible, a skilled and experienced operator should secure a definitive airway. This will both control and protect the airway and enable chest compressions to be given continuously, thus improving coronary perfusion. Once a definitive airway is established and compressions are uninterrupted, the ventilation rate should be 10–12 per minute. It is important for the team leader to assess that the ventilations remain adequate when chest compressions are continuous. This is most proficiently done by the person doing the chest compressions who can feel the chest moving when ventilated. The protocol for asystole and PEA is shown in Figure 7.21.

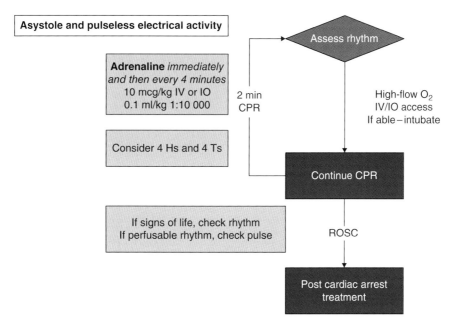

Figure 7.21 Protocol for asystole and pulseless electrical activity

During and following the administration of adrenaline, chest compressions and ventilations should continue. It is vital that chest compressions and ventilations continue uninterrupted during advanced life support as they form the basis of the resuscitative effort. The only reason to interrupt BLS is to shock the patient if needed and to check the rhythm. It may be necessary to briefly interrupt during difficult intubation.

At intervals of 2 minutes briefly pause in the delivery of chest compressions to assess the rhythm on the monitor. If asystole remains, continue CPR while again checking the electrode position and contacts. If there is an organised rhythm, check for signs of life and for a pulse. If there a return of spontaneous circulation (ROSC), continue post-resuscitation care, increasing ventilations to 12–24 breaths per minute according to age. If there are no signs of life and no pulse continue the protocol. Give adrenaline every 4 minutes at a dose of 10 micrograms/kg.

Reversible causes

Continually during CPR consider and correct reversible causes of the cardiac arrest based on the history of the event, known underlying illness in the child and any clues that are found during resuscitation. The causes of cardiac arrest in infancy and childhood are multifactorial but the two commonest pathways are through hypoxia and hypovolaemia.

All factors are conveniently remembered as the 4 Hs and 4 Ts:

- **H**ypoxia is a prime cause of cardiac arrest in childhood and is key to successful resuscitation
- **H**ypovolaemia may be significant in arrests associated with trauma, anaphylaxis and sepsis and requires infusion of crystalloid (see Section 6.10)
- **H**yperkalaemia, hypokalaemia, hypocalcaemia and other metabolic abnormalities may be suggested by the patient's underlying condition (e.g. renal failure), tests taken during the resuscitation or clues given in the ECG (Figure 7.22). Intravenous calcium (0.3 ml/kg of 10% calcium gluconate) is indicated in hyperkalaemia, hypocalcaemia and calcium channel blocker overdose
- **H**ypothermia is associated with drowning incidents and requires particular care
- **T**ension pneumothorax and cardiac **T**amponade are especially associated with PEA and are found in trauma cases.
- **T**oxic substances either as a result of accidental or deliberate overdose or from an iatrogenic mistake may require specific antidotes
- **T**hromboembolic phenomena are rare events in children but should still be considered

(a) Peaked T waves in hyperkalaemia ECG

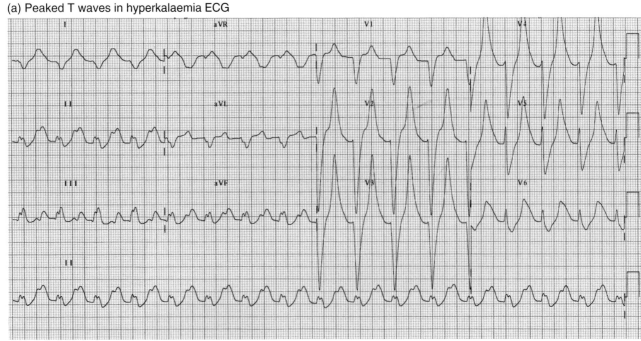

(b) Broad abnormal QRS in hyperkalaemia

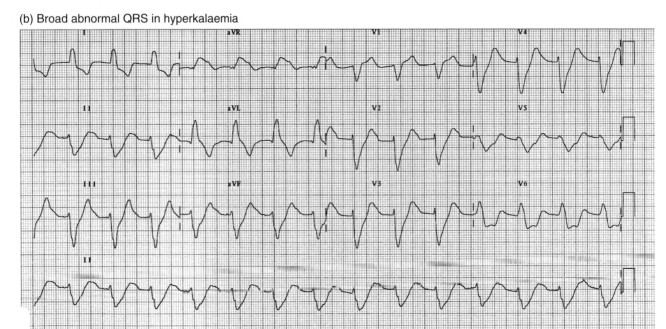

Figure 7.22 ECG changes in hyperkalaemia. Source: lifeinthefastlane.com

Adrenaline dosage

Adrenaline has been used for many years although its place has never been subjected to trial against placebo in children. In adults one prospective randomised study of drugs, including adrenaline, showed an improvement in ROSC but no increase in long-term neurologically intact survival. Another study with adrenaline against placebo showed similar results, but the number of patients was too low to make significant changes. The use of adrenaline is supported by animal studies and its known effects in improving relative coronary and cerebral perfusion. There was a trend to the use of higher doses of adrenaline in past years but evidence now links high dosage to poorer outcome, especially in asphyxial arrests. High-dose (100 micrograms/kg) adrenaline should only be used in very specific circumstances, e.g. if necessary after cardiac arrest associated with β-blocker overdose.

Alkalising agents

Children with asystole will be acidotic as cardiac arrest has usually been preceded by respiratory arrest or shock. However, the routine use of alkalising agents has not been shown to be of benefit. Sodium bicarbonate therapy increases intracellular carbon dioxide levels so administration, if used at all, should follow assisted ventilation with oxygen and effective BLS. Once ventilation is ensured and adrenaline plus chest compressions are provided to maximise circulation, use of sodium bicarbonate may be considered for the patient with prolonged cardiac arrest. These agents should be administered only in cases where profound acidosis is likely to adversely affect the action of adrenaline. In addition, sodium bicarbonate is recommended in the treatment of patients with hyperkalaemia and tricyclic antidepressant overdose.

In the arrested patient, arterial pH does not correlate well with tissue pH. Mixed venous or central venous pH should be used to guide any further alkalising therapy and it should always be remembered that good BLS is more effective than alkalising agents at raising myocardial pH.

Bicarbonate is the most common alkalising agent currently available, the dose being 1 mmol/kg (1 ml/kg of an 8.4% solution). If it must be used:

- Bicarbonate must not be given in the same intravenous line as calcium because precipitation will occur
- Sodium bicarbonate inactivates adrenaline and dopamine and therefore the line must be flushed with saline if these drugs are subsequently given
- Bicarbonate must not be given by the intratracheal route

Calcium

In the past, calcium was recommended in the treatment of PEA and asystole, but there is no evidence for its efficacy and there is evidence for harmful effects as calcium is implicated in cytoplasmic calcium accumulation in the final common pathway of cell death. This results from calcium entering cells following ischaemia and during reperfusion of ischaemic organs. Administration of calcium in the resuscitation of asystolic patients is not recommended. Calcium is indicated only for treatment of documented hypocalcaemia and hyperkalaemia, and for the treatment of hypermagnesaemia and of calcium channel blocker overdose. Dose 0.2 ml/kg of 10% calcium chloride.

Atropine

Atropine has no place in the management of cardiac arrest. Its use is to combat excessive vagal tone causing bradycardia in the perfusing patient and as an antidote in some poisonings.

7.7 Shockable rhythms

This includes ventricular fibrillation (VF) and pulseless ventricular tachycardia (pVT). ECGs showing VF and pVT are given in Figures 7.23 and 7.24, respectively.

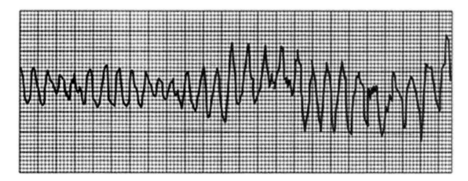

Figure 7.23 Ventricular fibrillation

These arrhythmias are less common in children but either may be expected in sudden collapse, in those suffering from hypothermia, in poisoning by tricyclic antidepressants and in those with cardiac disease. The protocol for VF and pVT is the same and is shown in Figure 7.25.

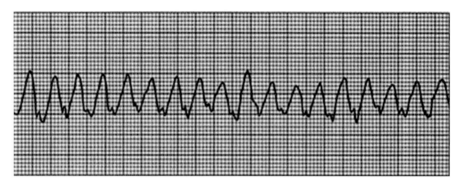

Figure 7.24 Pulseless ventricular tachycardia

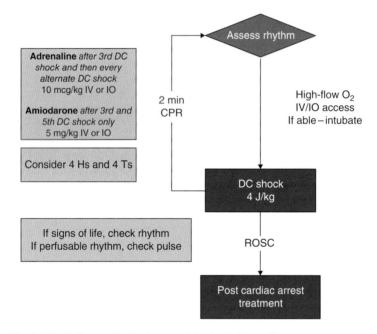

Figure 7.25 Protocol for ventricular fibrillation and pulseless ventricular tachycardia

There is little direct evidence for the best approach to cardiac arrest from VF/pVT in children. The guidance is based on that developed for adults, although it is recognised that the pathology causing VF/pVT arrest in children is both less common and more varied than that in adults. Recognised causes of VF/pVT in children include underlying cardiac disease, usually congenital, hypothermia and some drug overdoses. A sudden witnessed collapse is also suggestive of a VF/pVT episode.

If the patient is being monitored, the rhythm can be identified before significant deterioration. With immediate identification of VF/pVT, asynchronous electrical defibrillation of 4 joules per kilogram (J/kg) should be carried out immediately and the protocol continued as below.

In unmonitored children, BLS will have been started in response to the collapse and the identification of VF/pVT will occur when the cardiac monitor is put in place.

An asynchronous shock of 4 J/kg should be given straight away and CPR immediately resumed without reassessing the rhythm or feeling for a pulse. Immediate resumption of CPR is vital because there is a pause between successful defibrillation and the appearance of a rhythm on the monitor. Cessation of chest compressions will reduce the chance of a successful outcome if a further shock is needed. No harm accrues from 'unnecessary' compressions.

Appropriately sized adhesive defibrillation pads should be used. Recommended sizes are 4.5 cm for children <10 kg and 8–12 cm for children >10 kg. One pad is placed over the apex in the mid-axillary line, whilst the other is put immediately below the clavicle just to the right of the sternum. If only adult pads are available or your pads are too large for the infant/child, one should be placed on the upper back, below the left scapula, and the other on the front, to the left of the sternum.

In the event of a neonate requiring defibrillation, commercially available paediatric pads are not sufficiently small enough.

If the shock fails to defibrillate, attention must revert to supporting coronary and cerebral perfusion as in asystole. Although the procedures to stabilise the airway and gain circulatory access are now described sequentially, they should be undertaken simultaneously under the direction of a resuscitation team leader.

The airway should be secured, the patient ventilated with high-flow oxygen and effective chest compressions continued at a rate of 100–120 per minute, a compression depth of at least one-third of the anteroposterior diameter of the chest or 4 cm for infants and by 5 cm for children at a ratio of 15 compressions to two ventilations. As soon as is feasible, a skilled and experienced operator should intubate the child's airway. This will both control and protect the airway and enable chest compressions to be given continuously, thus improving coronary perfusion. Once the child has been intubated and compressions are uninterrupted, the ventilation rate should be 10–12 per minute. It is important for the team leader to assess that the ventilations remain adequate when chest compressions are continuous. Gain circulatory access. Whenever venous access is not attainable within 1 minute, intraosseous access should be used as it is rapid and effective. In each case any drug is followed by a normal saline flush (2–5 ml).

- Two minutes after the first shock, pause the chest compressions briefly to check the monitor. If VF/pVT is still present, give a second shock of 4 J/kg and immediately resume CPR, commencing with chest compressions
- Consider and correct reversible causes (4 Hs and 4 Ts) while continuing CPR for a further 2 minutes. Pause briefly to check the monitor
- If the rhythm is still VF/pVT give a third shock of 4 J/kg

Resume chest compressions immediately and, once established, give adrenaline 10 micrograms/kg and amiodarone 5 mg/kg IV or IO, flushing after each drug. After completion of the 2 minutes of CPR, pause briefly to check the monitor and if the rhythm is still VF/pVT give an immediate fourth shock of 4 J/kg and resume CPR.

After a further 2 minutes of CPR, pause briefly to check the monitor and if the rhythm is still shockable, give an immediate fifth shock of 4 J/kg.

Resume chest compressions immediately and, once established, give a second dose of adrenaline 10 micrograms/kg and a second dose of amiodarone 5 mg/kg IV or IO.

After completion of the 2 minutes of CPR pause briefly before the next shock to check the monitor.

Continue giving shocks every 2 minutes, minimising the pauses in CPR as much as possible. Give adrenaline after every alternate shock (i.e. every 4 minutes) and continue to seek and treat reversible causes.

Note: after each 2 minutes of uninterrupted CPR, pause briefly to assess the rhythm on the monitor for no more than 5 seconds. In addition, if at any time there are signs of life, such as regular respiratory effort, coughing, eye opening or a sudden increase in end-tidal CO_2 (see below) stop CPR and check the monitor:

- If still VF/pVT, continue with the sequence as above
- If asystole, change to the asystole/PEA giving adrenaline every 4 minutes
- If organised electrical activity is seen, check for signs of life and a pulse; if there is ROSC, continue post resuscitation care. If there is no pulse (or a pulse below 60 beats per minute with no signs of circulation and poor perfusion) and no other signs of life continue the asystole/PEA sequence.

Antiarrhythmic drugs

Amiodarone is the treatment of choice in shock-resistant VF and pVT. This is based on evidence from adult cardiac arrest and experience with the use of amiodarone in children in the catheterisation laboratory setting. The dose of amiodarone for VF/pVT is 5 mg/kg via rapid intravenous bolus.

In VF/pVT caused by an overdose of an arrhythmogenic drug, the use of amiodarone should be omitted. Expert advice should be obtained from a poisons centre. Amiodarone is likely to be unhelpful in the setting of VF caused by hypothermia but may be used, nevertheless.

Lidocaine (lignocaine) is an alternative to amiodarone if the latter is unavailable. The dose is 1 mg/kg IV or IO. It is the DC shock that converts the heart back to a perfusing rhythm, not the drug. The purpose of the antiarrhythmic drug is to stabilise the converted rhythm and the purpose of adrenaline is to improve myocardial oxygenation by increasing coronary perfusion pressure. Adrenaline also increases the vigour and intensity of ventricular fibrillation, which increases the success of defibrillation.

Magnesium 25–50 mg/kg (maximum of 2 g) is indicated in children with hypomagnesaemia or with polymorphic ventricular tachycardia (torsades de pointes), regardless of cause.

Reversible causes

During CPR consider and correct reversible causes of the cardiac arrest based on the history of the event and any clues that are found during resuscitation.

These factors are remembered as the 4 Hs and 4 Ts (see full list earlier in the chapter).

If there is still resistance to defibrillation, different paddle positions or another defibrillator may be tried. In the infant in whom paediatric paddles have been used, larger paddles applied to the front and back of the chest may be an alternative.

If the rhythm initially converts and then deteriorates back to VF or pVT then the sequence should continue to cycle, omitting a further dose of amiodarone if two doses have already been given. If further amiodarone is thought necessary, an infusion should be given of 300 micrograms/kg/h to a maximum of 1.5 mg/kg/h to a maximum of 1.2 g in 24 hours.

Automatic external defibrillators

The introduction of AEDs in the pre-hospital setting and especially for public access has significantly improved the outcome for VF/pVT cardiac arrest in adults in some settings. In the pre-hospital setting, AEDs are commonly used in adults to assess cardiac rhythm and to deliver defibrillation. Many AEDs can detect VF/pVT in children of all ages and differentiate 'shockable' from 'non-shockable' rhythms with a high degree of sensitivity and specificity. Thus, if an AED is the only defibrillator available, its use should be considered (preferably with the paediatric pads) as described earlier.

These devices have paediatric attenuation pads that decrease the energy to a level more appropriate for the child (1–8 years) or leads reducing the total energy to 50–80 joules. For the infant of less than 1 year, a manual defibrillator that can be adjusted to give the correct shock is recommended. However, if an AED is the only defibrillator available, its use should be considered, preferably with paediatric attenuation pads. The order of decreasing preference for defibrillation in the under 1-year-olds is as follows:

1. Manual defibrillator
2. AED with dose attenuator
3. AED without dose attenuator

Modern defibrillators now use biphasic wave forms. Defibrillation appears to be as effective at lower energy doses as conventional wave forms in adults and the energy appears to cause less myocardial damage than monophasic shocks. Both monophasic and biphasic wave form defibrillators are acceptable for use in childhood.

Capnography

Monitoring of end-tidal CO_2 ($ETCO_2$) can be helpful in managing cardiac arrest as long as the operator appreciates that the absence of a waveform is more likely to be due to absent or very poor pulmonary perfusion than to tube misplacement. The presence of exhaled CO_2 during CPR is encouraging evidence of efficacy of CPR or even ROSC. Adrenaline will decrease and bicarbonate increase the measured CO_2. Levels of less than 2 kPa (15 mmHg) should prompt attention to chest compression adequacy.

Oxygen use

While 100% oxygen, when available, remains the recommendation for use during the resuscitation process outside the delivery room, once there is ROSC there can be damage to recovering tissues from hyperoxia. Pulse oximetry should be used to monitor and adjust for oxygen requirement after a successful resuscitation. Saturations should then be maintained between 94% and 98%.

Hypoglycaemia

All children, especially infants, can become hypoglycaemic when seriously ill. Blood glucose should be checked frequently and hypoglycaemia corrected carefully. It is important not to cause hyperglycaemia as this will promote an osmotic diuresis. Both hypoglycaemia and hyperglycaemia are associated with a worse neurological outcome in animal models of cardiac arrest.

7.8 Traumatic cardiorespiratory arrest

Traumatic cardiorespiratory arrest (TCRA) is not an unsurvivable event and survival rates in literature are as high as 25% in selected populations. However, it requires rapid, aggressive and coordinated treatment to achieve a successful outcome. It is the pinnacle of pre-hospital trauma management teamwork. The management of TCRA is different to the management of cardiac arrest secondary to illness.

Causes of TCRA

- Hypoxia (following primary apnoea in head injury or airway obstruction)
- Hypovolaemia
- Tension pneumothorax
- Cardiac tamponade
- High spinal injury

The identification of arrest may be difficult in extremely low cardiac output states but the management is the same. The cause of arrest may be difficult to identify thus the algorithm in Figure 7.26 should be applied. The first three steps should be performed in all cases of TCRA, concurrently if resources allow. Once they have been achieved, a rapid assessment and consideration of the need to perform a thoracotomy should occur (if trained).

Thoracotomy

Many pre-hospital critical care teams will have this capability. Outcomes in paediatric thoracotomy are similar to those in adults and its role in the management of penetrating trauma with TCRA is beyond doubt. The aim of thoracotomy is to release cardiac tamponade, gain control of pulmonary haemorrhage or enable proximal occlusion of the descending aorta.

Thoracotomy in blunt trauma or massive peripheral haemorrhage is becoming commoner in adult practice and although its role in paediatric practice is not yet quantified it is likely to emerge as a strategy in paediatric blunt trauma TCRA.

Cardiac compressions

External cardiac compressions are unlikely to be effective in traumatic cardiac arrest and should not be performed if doing so diverts effort from treating the causes of arrest. Once these have been addressed then compressions can be performed, particularly if filling has been achieved.

Adrenaline

Adrenaline is not indicated in traumatic arrest and should not be given. The exception to this is in the event of arrest secondary to high spinal injury to reverse loss of sympathetic tone.

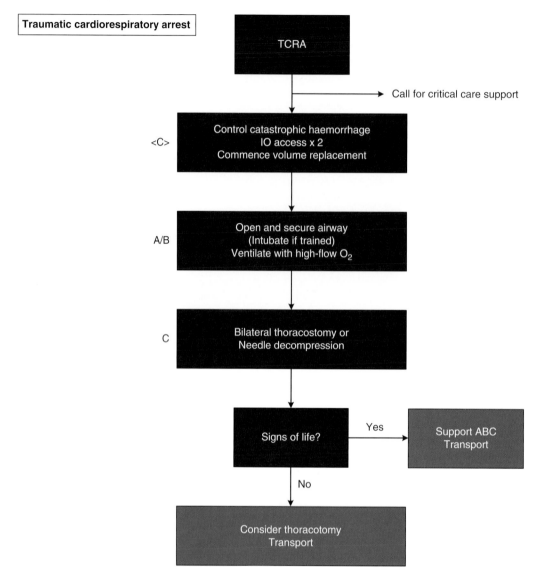

Figure 7.26 Traumatic cardiorespiratory arrest (TCRA) algorithm

7.9 Newborn resuscitation

Background

The resuscitation of newborn babies is different from the resuscitation of all other age groups and knowledge of the relevant physiology and pathophysiology is essential. However, the majority of newborn babies will establish normal respiration and circulation spontaneously.

After delivery of a healthy term baby, the first breath usually occurs within 60 seconds of clamping, or obstructing, the umbilical cord. Clamping of the cord leads to the onset of asphyxia, which is the major stimulant to start respiration. Physical stimuli, such as cold air or physical discomfort, help provoke respiratory efforts. The first breaths are especially important as the lungs are initially full of fluid.

Labour causes the cells within the lung that secrete lung fluid to cease secretion and begin reabsorption of that fluid. During vaginal delivery up to 35 ml of fluid is expelled from the baby's lungs by uterine contractions. In a healthy baby, the first spontaneous breaths generate a negative pressure of between −40 and −100 cmH$_2$O (−3.9 and −13 kPa), which inflate the lungs for the first time. This pressure is 10–15 times greater than that needed for later breathing, when the lungs are aerated, but is necessary to overcome the viscosity of fluid filling the airways, the surface tension of the fluid-filled lungs and the elastic recoil and resistance of the chest wall, lungs and airways and the resistance of the airways. These powerful chest movements cause fluid to be displaced from the airways into the lymphatics.

Acute asphyxia deprives the body of oxygen. Initially breathing becomes deeper and more rapid, and if unsuccessful the baby loses consciousness quite quickly; increasing hypoxia causes cessation of breathing within 2–3 minutes (primary apnoea). Babies have a number of automatic reflex responses to such a situation: energy is conserved by shutting down the circulation to all but the vital organs, such as the heart, lungs and brain. Bradycardia ensues but blood pressure is maintained by peripheral vasoconstriction and increased stroke volume.

After a latent period of primary apnoea, which may vary in duration, spinal gasps ensue. These deep spontaneous gasps are easily distinguishable from normal respirations as they occur 6–12 times per minute and involve all accessory muscles in a maximal inspiratory effort. After a while, even this activity ceases (terminal apnoea) and the most primitive medullary reflexes are extinguished. The time taken for such activity to cease is longer in the newborn than in later life, taking up to 20 minutes.

It is now recommended that well babies have a delay in having the cord cut as this will increase the infant's haemoglobin level. The umbilicus should remain at, or below, the level of the placenta for a minute, while keeping the baby warm. Evidence for doing this with compromised babies is not available, and in those needing resuscitation the priority remains to resuscitate.

What to look for

If the baby is a term baby and well, they will be pink, cry and breathe normally and have a heart rate above 100/minute.

All babies should be:

- Dried (unless they are less than 32 weeks' gestation, in which case they should be wrapped wet in food-grade cling film and provided with radiant heat if available, otherwise wrapped in dry towels)
- They can then be assessed while keeping them as warm as possible – the major priority in those born before getting to hospital
- Given to the mother if possible (skin to skin, or for a child in a plastic bag, placed against the mother's skin as this will help maintain body temperature)

If the baby is compromised they will fall into the category of those with primary or secondary apnoea (Table 7.2).

Table 7.2 Assessment of the newborn			
	Healthy	**Primary apnoea**	**Terminal apnoea**
Colour	Pink	Blue	Blue/white
Respiration	Regular	Irregular or inadequate	Absent
Heart rate	120–150/min	>100/min	<100/min

Management

Resuscitation consists of:

- Opening the airway
- Aerating the lungs (inflation breaths)
- Rescue breathing
- Chest compression
- Administration of drugs (rarely)

Babies that are less well or ill should have the following performed:

- The airway should be opened and cleared
- Five rescue breaths should be given with a bag and mask, preferably using room air
- Oxygen should NOT be used in this group initially
- If there is no improvement in heart rate or breathing, try altering the position of the airway; higher pressure inflation may be needed or the oropharynx may be obstructed
- If the chest is moving and the heart rate improves, keep ventilating at a rate of about 30–40 per minute (reassessing every 30 seconds) until the baby breathes on their own
- The heart rate must be assessed by listening over the heart with a stethoscope – peripheral pulses are unreliable in this situation

The vast majority of babies will respond to ventilations alone.

If the baby fails to respond rapidly to good ventilations:

- *Attach a pulse oximeter to the RIGHT hand of the baby (to measure pre-ductal arterial oxygen saturation or SpO_2)*

Acceptable pre-ductal SpO_2

2 minutes: 60%

3 minutes: 70%

4 minutes: 80%

5 minutes: 85%

10 minutes: 90%

- If oxygen levels are less than shown in the box above, adjust the oxygen flow to correct them. Try not to let levels get above 95%, particularly in the pre-term baby as high levels can be harmful
- If the chest wall is **moving well**, but the heart rate remains less than 60/minute, start chest compressions at a rate of 3:1

The best method is the 'encircling' method (Figure 7.27). Here, the baby's chest is gripped in both hands in such a way that the two thumbs can press on the lower third of the sternum, just below an imaginary line joining the nipples, with the fingers over the spine at the back. Compress **quickly and firmly**, depressing the chest wall by about one-third. Allow time for ventilations to inflate the chest and for the chest to recoil.

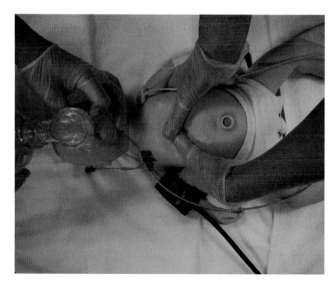

Figure 7.27 Hand-encircling technique for chest compressions

Reassess every 30 seconds – if not improving, consider venous access and drugs.

Less than 1:1000 babies will need drugs. There evidence in animal studies that adrenaline and bicarbonate may improve outcome, but in humans there is no placebo-controlled evidence showing that any drug will improve outcome.

Doses of drugs

- Adrenaline 10 micrograms/kg first dose, up to 30 micrograms/kg second dose
- Bicarbonate 1–2 mg/kg
- Dextrose 2.5 ml/kg 10% dextrose

When to stop

If there has been no detectable heart beat for at least 10 minutes, it is reasonable to consider discontinuing resuscitation. However, this may depend on the reason for the arrest and other factors including parental feelings regarding the eventual outcome for their child. This is a senior decision.

Notes

Suction and meconium

- There is no evidence that suctioning while the baby is on the perineum improves the outcome of meconium aspiration syndrome
- There is no evidence that intubating a vigorous baby with meconium-stained liquor improves the outcome of subsequent meconium aspiration syndrome
- It is reasonable to suction the oropharynx and endotracheal tube in a collapsed baby to remove meconium, but prolonged attempts at intubation should not be carried out as there is no convincing evidence of benefit
- There is no evidence to confirm or refute suction of babies without meconium, but if it is overvigorous it may cause bradycardia

Figure 7.28 summarises the procedure for the resuscitation of newborns.

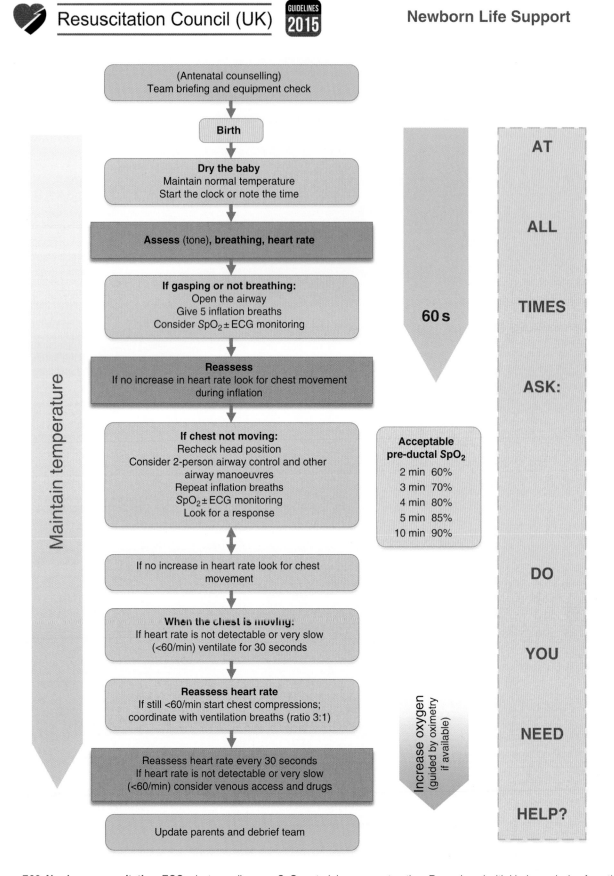

Figure 7.28 Newborn resuscitation. ECG, electrocardiogram; SpO_2, arterial oxygen saturation. Reproduced with kind permission from the Resuscitation Council (UK)

CHAPTER 8
When a child dies

Learning outcomes

After reading this chapter, you will be able to:
- Identify the factors that are important when dealing with the death of a child
- Describe your approach to the death of a child
- Identify your role in dealing with the death of a child
- Have an awareness of 'Do not attempt resuscitation' orders

8.1 Sudden death of a child

Even with the best preventative measures in place and the use of the most effective resuscitation methods, children will continue to die from serious illness and severe injury. This is particularly so in out-of-hospital cardiac arrest and in the case of sudden unexpected death of infants and children (SUDIC).

All those involved in pre-hospital care are likely to have to cope with the sudden death of a child. This can be very stressful to the staff involved, who have to deal not only with the parents or carers, but also with their own feelings. Those involved need to be supported in this aspect of their work by being taught about it beforehand and having the opportunity for counselling sessions afterwards.

Parental presence during cardiopulmonary resuscitation is now generally accepted practice, although parents should have the choice whether to be there or not. In an ideal situation a healthcare professional should be available exclusively for the support of the parents, but in most out-of-hospital situations this will not be practical because the same personnel will be doing both the resuscitation and supporting the parents.

If the child has been the victim of an accident and the injuries have resulted in disfigurement or deformity there is a natural tendency to try to prevent the parents from seeing their child. Usually parents can handle severe injuries. The uppermost thought in their minds is to be with their child, to hold his or her hand and to provide affection and comfort to the end of life. Many parents subsequently complain that they were overprotected by healthcare workers and regret that they were denied what they considered to be precious last moments with their child and the chance to say 'goodbye'.

If the decision that the child has died has been made and resuscitation is clearly inappropriate, then the parents should be told as soon as possible. The news should be broken sympathetically and without euphemisms, the language used should be wholly unambiguous. Sympathy and support can be shown by holding the parent's hand or by putting an arm around them, if it is felt appropriate. It is acceptable that even in the face of certain futility resuscitation can be started and continued during transport to hospital. This will provide support for both providers and parents when the decision to stop is made.

Pre-Hospital Paediatric Life Support: A Practical Approach to Emergencies, Third Edition. Edited by Alan Charters, Hal Maxwell and Paul Reavley.
© 2017 John Wiley & Sons Ltd. Published 2017 by John Wiley & Sons Ltd.

Most deaths in infancy and childhood are due to natural causes or accidents, but occasionally infanticide or homicide does occur. Careful notes should be made of any unusual circumstances in the home or at the scene from which the child was moved to hospital. This information may be very valuable to any investigation by the police on behalf of the coroner, who is always informed of sudden unexpected deaths.

In most cases, the child should be transported to the hospital even if they have been confirmed as dead. The reasons for this are that a full history, post-death investigations and proper counselling of the parents are essential and easier to arrange through the hospital. Inform the hospital of the expected time of arrival and whether resuscitation is being attempted. However, post-death procedure will vary from region to region, and country to country, so be aware of your working area's protocol.

During the journey to hospital, transport the child as you would a patient who is alive. The parents may wish to hold their baby. The parents should be allowed to help look after their child in the ambulance, even if resuscitation is in progress. Ensure that both parents or one parent and a relative or friend are available to support each other. Give advice on practical issues, such as the care of other children, locking the house and taking keys to the hospital. Be prepared to handle any reaction – silence, shouting, numbness and crying are all normal reactions to a suspicion or knowledge that a child is dead or dying. At all stages be very careful what you say to the parents. Chance remarks linger in the memory.

Be aware of any personal difficulties that you have in handling death and bereavement and consider support or counselling for this, preferably before another similar situation arises. Most ambulance services in the UK will have Trauma Risk Management (TRiM) practitioners to offer brief intervention following difficult cases like a child death.

In summary, the principles in dealing with a family that has experienced a sudden child death are shown in the box below.

Principles in dealing with a family

- Display caring, kindness and compassion
- Spend as much time as necessary with the family in an unhurried fashion
- Offer information regarding the death as the family requires
- Talk to colleagues later regarding your experience and feelings

---

8.2 Post-death procedures

Every jurisdiction will have specific legal requirements that need to be adhered to. It is usually necessary for the coroner, the police or another statutory authority to be informed of the death. The requirements for a police or coronial investigation, an autopsy and an inquest will vary from case to case.

Having a clear protocol for dealing with a child death will be invaluable for ensuring that procedures or information are not forgotten. Local hospital guidelines should be followed. In all cases of sudden unexpected death in the UK, there are local procedures for reporting to and investigation by a multi-agency team led by the Designated Doctor for Unexpected Deaths.

Dealing with death

The child

- Attempt cardiopulmonary resuscitation unless death is certain
- Transport the child on a stretcher or in the arms of a parent
- Always transport the child to hospital unless the police dictate otherwise for forensic reasons
- Always refer to the child by name and the appropriate gender
- Never put a child in a black body bag

The parents

- Explain that the child has died if qualified to say so
- Allow parents to be with their child if they so wish on the journey to hospital
- Allow two adults to accompany the child if practical
- Advise on the care of other children, locking the house, taking keys, etc.
- Always be gentle, unhurried, calm and careful in the words that you use
- Remember that many reactions in the acute stage of bereavement are normal

Yourself

- Inform the hospital of the expected time of arrival and whether resuscitation is being attempted
- Be aware of any personal difficulties you may have in handling the death of a child and obtain support beforehand and through staff counselling sessions afterwards

8.3 Do not attempt resuscitation orders

For a small number of children who suffer from terminal illness, death at home may be planned and expected. In such cases resuscitation would be entirely inappropriate. To avoid confusion it is helpful if the local ambulance service has processes in place for alerting crews of terminally ill patients so that crews are not put in the difficult position of undertaking procedures that are inappropriate and potentially very distressing for parents and carers. Though in most situations parents are unlikely to call for an ambulance, an unexpected event, such as a fit, or the child deteriorating while with an unfamiliar carer, may lead to a crew being summoned.

To address such an event the prior writing of a 'Do not attempt resuscitation' (DNAR) order, signed by the GP or consultant with medical responsibility for the child, and the parent, which is dated and written in such a way that the crew will recognise the authority, can avoid confusion and distress. You should be aware of the format of such orders, which are being requested with increasing frequency by carers of both children and adults.

CHAPTER 9
The non-seriously ill child

Learning outcomes

After reading this chapter, you will be able to:
- Describe your approach to the less seriously ill child
- Describe some of the common but not serious conditions of childhood

---

Assessment of illness in children can be challenging for the paediatrician and non-paediatrician alike. There are some basic principles that should be followed:

1. Make use of recognised assessment tools and guidelines that are readily understood by all clinicians dealing with the child. Examples include:
   - National Institute for Health and Care Excellence (NICE) Clinical Guideline 160 –*Fever in Under 5s: Assessment and Early Management* (May 2013). This is shown in Table 9.1
   - NICE Clinical Guideline 176 – *Head Injury: Assessment and Early Management* (January 2014)
   - British Thoracic Society/Scottish Intercollegiate Guidelines Network (SIGN) Quick Reference Guide 2014 – *British Guideline on the Management of Asthma* (October 2014)
2. Do not feel you have to cope alone. Access available advice and support
3. Never be afraid or embarrassed to discuss a child with the hospital or someone more senior or to send a child into hospital for further assessment
4. Trust your gut feelings – never walk away from a child feeling uncomfortable about the level of treatment you have provided or decisions you have made
5. Communicate your decision to the parents or carers and support it with clear explanation; offer written information if possible
6. Make provision for a 'safety net' taking into account factors that indicate a need for further review and/or admission to hospital. Make it absolutely clear when further medical advice should be sought and, again, if possible leave written notes. For example:
   - Child has had a fit
   - Poor oral intake/poor feeding
   - Drowsiness/irritability
   - Child has developed a non-blanching rash
   - Parent or carer feels that the child is less well than when they previously sought advice or the child is failing to improve
   - Parent or carer is more worried than when they previously sought advice
   - Fever has lasted longer than 5 days
   - Parent or carer is distressed, or concerned that they are unable to look after their child

---

Pre-Hospital Paediatric Life Support: A Practical Approach to Emergencies, Third Edition. Edited by Alan Charters, Hal Maxwell and Paul Reavley.
© 2017 John Wiley & Sons Ltd. Published 2017 by John Wiley & Sons Ltd.

Table 9.1 Traffic light system for identifying risk of serious illness

	Green – low risk	Amber – intermediate risk	Red – high risk
Colour (of skin, lips or tongue)	• Normal colour	• Pallor reported by parent/carer	• Pale/mottled/ashen/blue
Activity	• Responds normally to social cues • Content/smiles • Stays awake or awakens quickly • Strong normal cry/not crying	• Not responding normally to social cues • No smile • Wakes only with prolonged stimulation • Decreased activity	• No response to social cues • Appears ill to a healthcare professional • Does not wake or if roused does not stay awake • Weak, high-pitched or continuous cry
Respiratory		• Nasal flaring • Tachypnoea: – RR > 50 breaths/minute, age 6–12 months – RR > 40 breaths/minute, age > 12 months • Oxygen saturation ≤ 95% in air • Crackles in the chest	• Grunting • Tachypnoea: RR > 60 breaths/minute • Moderate or severe chest indrawing
Circulation and hydration	• Normal skin and eyes • Moist mucous membranes	• Tachycardia: – > 160 beats/minute, age < 12 months – > 150 beats/minute, age 12–24 months – > 140 beats/minute, age 2–5 years • CRT ≥ 3 seconds • Dry mucous membranes • Poor feeding in infants • Reduced urine output	• Reduced skin turgor
Other	• None of the amber or red symptoms or signs	• Age 3–6 months temperature ≥ 39°C • Fever for ≥ 5 days • Rigors • Swelling of a limb or joint • Non-weight-bearing limb/not using an extremity	• Age < 3 months, temperature ≥ 38°C • Non-blanching rash • Bulging fontanelle • Neck stiffness • Status epilepticus • Focal neurological signs • Focal seizures

This traffic light table should be used in conjuction with the recommendations in the guideline on investigations and initial management in children with fever.
Source: National Institute for Health and Care Excellence (2013) *CG160 Fever in Under 5's: Assessment and Early Management*. Manchester: NICE. Available from www.nice.org.uk/CG160. Reproduced with permission of NICE.

Once the decision has been made that a child is not seriously ill and does not require admission, the pre-hospital practitioner is then required to implement a management plan. In some ways this can be more of a challenge than taking the decision to transport a child to hospital.

Rather than being a comprehensive paediatric text, this book is designed to offer practical advice as to how to deal with sick children for whom the carers have requested help. To this end, some of the commoner situations and illnesses are presented below, along with some notes, which may be helpful. The list of problems is not exhaustive and neither are the solutions. Of course there will be children who require hospital admission for relatively trivial illness and maybe more judgement calls have to be made when assessing a less seriously ill child than in managing a child in a life-threatening state.

Of particular importance may be:

- The degree of anxiety, experience and maturity of the parents or carers. This is coloured by the previous experience of the carers themselves or their friends and family as well as factors like the availability of support and advice
- The distance from hospital or help
- The ease of access for reviewing the child. Review can be by telephone in some cases but this is usually only appropriate when you either know the patient and their carers or have previously seen and assessed the child
- The social circumstances – including other children, etc.
- Previous medical history
- Presence of chronic illness (see Chapter 10)
- Previous medical experiences in this or other illnesses. This includes both yourself as the healthcare professional and the parents/carers
- The number of times that help has been sought for this episode. If you are asked to see the same child a second time ask yourself what has changed and/or what you have missed – it may be something about the child who is ill or may also be something about the parents/carers experience of which you have not been aware
- If asked to see the child a third time seriously consider admission to hospital for further opinion and advice
- The time of day – or night
- The confidence and experience that you as the *healthcare professional* have

Table 9.2 provides the signs and symptoms of common presentations in children in the absence of serious findings and discusses the treatment and disposition of these conditions. Also shown against some of the conditions are 'red flags', i.e. pointers to a more serious situation where further action should be considered. One red flag that should be considered is the presence of an underlying chronic condition that makes it more difficult for the child to cope with what may otherwise be relatively mild symptoms, e.g. mild upper respiratory symptoms can be life threatening in a child with a muscular dystrophy.

Table 9.2 Common childhood illnesses not requiring hospital admission and their treatment and disposition

Condition	Symptoms	Signs	Plan	Disposition	Red flags
Upper respiratory tract infection	• Cough • 'Cold' • Sore throat • Snuffly • Hot and miserable • Off food	• Inflamed throat • Running or stuffy nose • Chest clear	Symptomatic treatment	Care at home	• Poor or no oral intake • Less urine output or fewer wet nappies than is normal for the child
Conjunctivitis	• Sore, gritty eyes • Normal visual acuity	• Mildly inflamed conjunctiva • Sometimes purulent discharge	Good hygiene Antibiotic eye drops	Care at home	Painful eye Pain on eye movement Visual loss
Foreign body in nose, ear or throat	• History of witnessed insertion of object in nose or ear • 'Missing' object • Choking • Coughing	• Foreign body visible • Potentially, stridor • Consider also if unilateral nasal or ear discharge	May be possible to remove – if not refer to appropriate specialist	Care at home if object removed, otherwise refer to ED or appropriate specialist	Pain Respiratory distress Stridor Wheeze Cough
Tonsillitis	• Sore throat • Systemically unwell • Sore neck • Difficulty swallowing	• Swollen inflamed tonsils • Lymphadenopathy • Fever possible • May be exudates	Mild – symptomatic treatment; otherwise antibiotic and symptomatic treatment	Care at home with advice to recall if upper airway becomes noisy	• Peritonsillar redness and swelling • Inadequate oral intake • Stridor
Teething	• Miserable	• Teeth erupting	Symptomatic treatment	Care at home	
Otitis media	• Miserable	• Inflamed ear drum ± perforation • Fever possible	Symptomatic treatment; consider antibiotics if very severe or eardrum is perforated	Care at home; consider non-urgent referral if infection is recurrent and severe or if ear drum is perforated	Mastoid tenderness Auricular cellulitis
Fever Fever is a sign, not a diagnosis – cause must be sought and found	• Hot • Off food/fluids	• Depend on cause	Exclude serious causes, e.g.: • severe sepsis • meningitis • meningococcal septicaemia • appendicitis • UTI Give symptomatic treatment and do not give antibiotics if cause unknown	Care at home; refer to hospital if cause cannot be identified or is potentially serious	As per Table 9.1 above

Condition	Symptoms	Clinical signs	Treatment	Management	Warning signs
Croup (mild) Clinical signs present when upset or active but are not present at rest	• Barking cough • Cough • SOB	• Barking cough • May have mild stridor • Child not distressed • Mild fever possible	Nebulised budesonide or oral dexamethasone or soluble prednisolone	Care at home with instructions to seek help if condition deteriorates	Signs of respiratory distress Signs of sepsis
Asthma (mild)	• Wheeze • Cough • May be URTI	• Bilateral wheeze • Good air entry • Mild tachypnoea • Child not distressed	Adjustment of dose of bronchodilator – multidosing approach, i.e. 10 puffs of inhaler via spacer. Check technique of administration using spacer. Oral (soluble) prednisolone	Care at home	Signs of severe or life-threatening asthma (see Chapter 5)
Bronchiolitis (mild)	• URTI followed by respiratory symptoms • 'Chesty' wheeze • Cough	• Not distressed • Mild tachypnoea • Mild fever possible • Bilateral fine crackles and wheeze	Symptomatic treatment	Care at home with instructions to seek help if condition deteriorates	• Reduced feeds • Dehydration • Pallor/cyanosis • Respiratory distress • Apnoeas
Chicken pox (uncomplicated)	• Mild URTI symptoms • Rash	• Blistering rash in crops, most marked on trunk • Mild fever possible	Symptomatic treatment	Care at home	Second episode of fever (secondary infection) Cellulitis
Scabies	• Itchy rash	• Itchy papules, may be more generalised than in adults, with some 'tracks'	Non-urgent referral to GP	Care at home and non-urgent referral to GP	
Impetigo	• Crusting rash	• Yellow/golden crusting, spreading rash • May be systemically unwell	Systemic antibiotics unless very tiny lesion when topical antibiotics may be tried	Care at home Advise on reducing spread to other family members	Signs of sepsis
Increase in seizures in child known to have seizures			Look for infection, recent change in medication dose or not taking medication or malabsorbing (e.g. GI upset) or any obvious cause If no cause found refer to GP or hospital as necessary	Refer to GP if not currently seizing and frequency of fits is acceptable and manageable	Atypical features Fever Rash Not recovering
Diarrhoea	Need description – ?blood ?slime ?amount	• No abdominal abnormalities • No signs of dehydration • No other sign of infection • May be mild fever	Encourage clear fluid intake Exclude occult infection and dehydration Refer small children who are very unwell or have bloody diarrhoea Exclude other abdominal pathology	Care at home; GP follow up if not resolving	Poor intake Dehydration

(Continued)

Table 9.2 (*Continued*)

Condition	Symptoms	Signs	Plan	Disposition	Red flags
Vomiting Note vomiting may be result of simple viral illness but may be a symptom of more serious illness	• Frequency • ?Blood • ?Tolerating clear fluids	• Not dehydrated • No other sign of infection	Exclude abdominal or other serious pathology If tolerating clear fluids, encourage clear fluids until improving, then solid diet **Consider sepsis**	Care at home, *unless red flags present*	• Bilious–green vomiting • Unwell or dehydrated or significant pathology cannot be excluded • Haematemisis
Febrile convulsion	• Fever, child known to have febrile convulsions • Age 6 months – 6 years	• Careful search for focus of infection and cause definitely found	Locate source of infection and treat, referring to hospital if serious cause found, or if *no* cause found Check blood sugar	Care at home for simple febrile convulsions, *unless red flags present*	• This is the first fit • The cause of the fever has not been identified • More than one fit in a 24-hour period • Prolonged seizure • Post-ictal • Focal seizure
Urinary tract infection	• Complaining of pain when passing urine • Frequency • Incontinence	• Positive urine analysis • Abdominal tenderness • Sepsis	Oral antibiotics Urine culture GP follow up	GP review Hospital review if red flags Referral to secondary care if recurrent or atypical infection is present	Back/loin pain Signs of sepsis
Headache	• Consider onset of headache • Symptoms of raised intracranial pressure	Lock for signs of: • Sepsis • Meningism	Simple analgesia	GP review if it persists *Referral if red flags present*	Sudden onset Persistent Photophobia Neck stiffness Postural features Vomiting Visual loss/change Focal neurology Morning exacerbation Papilloedema

CHAPTER 10
The chronically ill child

Learning outcomes

After reading this chapter, you will be able to:
- Describe how to make use of the parents' and patient's understanding of their illness and involve them in your management
- Describe the issues with some chronic illnesses in children that you may encounter

10.1 Introduction

Increasing numbers of children are now being treated for and surviving conditions that they would have previously not survived. Complex conditions require complex care requirements which depend on modern medical technology and pharmacology becoming part of the daily routine in their homes. Parents and carers develop a high level of knowledge of the particular condition and its management which is beyond that of most clinicians.

These dedicated families have enormous needs, worries and pressures and they can also present a significant challenge to a pre-hospital practitioner. They can certainly appear quite daunting to the health professional unless one remembers a few simple guidelines. The families and the pre-hospital care provider can work well together for the child's benefit with the guidance below.

Parents

1. LISTEN to what parents have to say. They may know much more about their child's emergency than you do. If what they say, however, does not appear to make sense, do not ignore it, but always clarify the situation with the hospital.
2. Ask if they have a summary of the child's condition and a written protocol from the hospital regarding what to do in an emergency.
3. Ask if they have a specialist nurse or similar who can be contacted for advice.
4. Resuscitation situations are often the usual management of ABC, BUT if the parents, or a written protocol, advise you otherwise, bear this in mind – contact the hospital or specialist unit urgently if you are not sure what to do.
5. Remember that parents may have a huge amount of knowledge regarding their child's long-term problem but that these children also get all the other problems that other children may have. The parents will not necessarily know any more about these 'normal' conditions than anybody else. This may be difficult to remember when they appear very expert. Ask them what is different about their child today.
6. Parents may have reactions you find disconcerting. They will be just as frightened of losing their child as anybody else, but may cope with the situation less well if they are already very stressed from looking after the child day in and day out. Alternatively, they may have been told a number of times that their child is unlikely to survive certain situations but the child has always done so. It can be very difficult to convince some parents that their child's life may be at threat this time when it has never happened before. A caring and professional manner will always be the best approach.
7. Parents do not want you to hurt or harm their child. If they tell you a child has a particularly good vein for venepuncture take their advice. The same goes for other simple procedures, which they may have witnessed may times.

Pre-Hospital Paediatric Life Support: A Practical Approach to Emergencies, Third Edition. Edited by Alan Charters, Hal Maxwell and Paul Reavley.
© 2017 John Wiley & Sons Ltd. Published 2017 by John Wiley & Sons Ltd.

The child

1. Children become expert at a very young age if they have grown up with a problem.
2. Like parents, they may know far more about their condition than many doctors. They will also have acute social awareness of their condition. Their insight is, however, age dependent. To an extent this depends on their peer group and social behaviour as well, and their knowledge and interest will be similarly biased. A tiny child will tell you what he is and is not allowed to eat, but will not necessarily have the social independence and peer influences to find out what happens if he or she breaks the rules, so may be relatively easy to manage. A teenager, in contrast, may rebel and experiment despite having more understanding and insight.

Some conditions are truly rare and even many paediatricians may not have heard of them. It is no loss of face, and may be essential to the child's best care, to ask the parents what exactly syndrome 'X' is. They will usually be able to provide information or, at a minimum, tell you who the child's specialist is. Encourage the parents to get the specialist to write a protocol for the child to be used in times of emergency, with a brief explanation of the condition.

10.2 Examples of complicated conditions you may encounter

Congenital heart disease

These children may present suddenly with circulatory collapse and shock, hypoxia or respiratory failure. Abnormalities can be very complex and sudden inadequate pulmonary or systemic blood may occur. The ductus arteriosus (a blood vessel linking the aorta and pulmonary circulation used in normal foetal circulation) will stay open for a while after birth to allow the baby to survive in certain severe abnormalities. Eventually, it starts to close and this may unmask a hitherto unknown life-threatening problem (this may occur up to a few weeks of age). These babies present with sudden, severe circulatory failure of unexplained cause and immediate transportation to a paediatric centre where they can be treated may be life saving. The main differential diagnosis is sepsis. Treat as per the shock algorithm (see Figure 5.3) and transfer urgently.

If a child with a known heart problem is blue, or has very low oxygen saturations, ask the parents what level of oxygen saturation is normal for them; parents will very often be able to tell you. Provide supplemental oxygen if saturations are below this.

Children with heart disease should only be given intravenous fluids cautiously and in no more than 5 ml/kg boluses with continuous reassessment of response. In the event of deterioration, the fluid should be discontinued even if this is only a slight deterioration.

As cardiovascular status can be difficult to assess clinically in congenital heart disease, if in any doubt transfer to secondary care for more detailed assessment and investigation.

Oncology

Cancer, particularly leukaemia is not uncommon in children and children may become ill at home while receiving active treatment, such as chemotherapy. Most of these children will have a central line to enable regular intravenous therapy. Like adults they may be severely immunosuppressed, and any fever in a child on chemotherapy will need specialist consultation and the measurement of a white cell count to exclude neutropenic sepsis. Parents will often monitor symptoms at home and have direct access to paediatric oncology advice via a nurse specialist or oncology centre. Other complications of chemotherapy and radiotherapy may occur and, again, parents may be vigilant for these.

Not all children have previously been exposed to or have received vaccination for certain viral infections, such as chicken pox or measles, and given their immunosuppressed state these can be life threatening. In the event of contact with these infections, the specialist unit must be informed urgently so that immunoglobulin may be given if necessary.

Transplant recipients

Liver, renal, heart and heart–lung transplants are all routinely performed in children in the UK. The anti-rejection drugs used may be heavily immunosuppressive and the same precautions as for oncology patients should generally be observed. Some anti-rejection drugs interact badly with fairly 'normal' primary care drugs (erythromycin and ciclosporin is a good example).

This group of children should only have medications prescribed by those with knowledge about the interactions of anti-rejection therapy and even then it is wise to check the *British National Formulary for Children (BNFc)* for up-to-date information and seek advice from a specialist pharmacist.

Renal disease

Children with renal conditions, including those on dialysis, may also sometimes be heavily immunosuppressed, with the problems and caveats in treatment as mentioned above.

Problems with dialysis lines are described in Table 10.1.

This group of children may be on very specialised diets and may have severe fluid restriction or massively increased requirements.

Children who are dialysis dependent will have raised urea, creatinine and potassium as they approach their dialysis appointment. In the presence of acute illness, this may be suddenly worse and hyperkalaemia in particular can be acutely life threatening. An electrocardiogram may show acute changes, widened QRS complexes and peaked T-waves.

Hypertension including hypertensive encephalopathy and convulsions may occur in children with renal disease.

Any fluid given in resuscitation should be titrated to response and the minimum amount to stabilise the child used (give 5 ml/kg aliquots with continuous reassessment of response).

Breathlessness may be due to pulmonary oedema due to fluid overload in children with renal disease and is a pre-terminal condition. Such children should be given oxygen but not given fluid unless it is certain the child is not fluid overloaded. Specialist advice will be helpful.

Ventilated children and those with tracheostomies

A number of children in the UK are on home ventilation, usually for central nervous system conditions or neuromuscular conditions, and will have tracheostomies. Tracheostomies may also be needed to circumvent upper airway conditions, e.g. laryngomalacia following prolonged ventilation such as in neonatal intensive care. Emergency tracheostomy care is outlined in Table 10.1.

Patients may deteriorate in the following situations:

- Equipment failure
- Lower respiratory tract infection
- Obstruction or displacement of the tracheostomy
- Secretions/lower airway collapse

Never take on the responsibility of a ventilator unless you have been trained to use it. Allow the trained carer to accompany the child and continue to look after the machine.

Diabetic ketoacidosis

Children with relatively insufficient insulin for their requirements are unable to metabolise sugar properly and will develop alternative, less effective methods of metabolism, which result in ketone production and acidosis. The high blood sugars encountered in this condition cause an osmotic diuresis leading to dehydration and if this occurs relatively rapidly, shock, as fluid is also lost from the intravascular compartment. Thus the usual story of a new or out of control diabetic is one of thirst, polyuria and weight loss and eventually drowsiness. The acidosis eventually becomes sufficiently severe that the respiratory compensation may be obvious with tachypnoea. It is relatively unusual for children with diabetic ketoacidosis to require resuscitation pre-hospital, but if they are very drowsy, oxygen should be given, and if shocked, the shock should also be addressed.

Note that IV fluids should be given more slowly in diabetic ketoacidosis because these children are prone to cerebral oedema; dehydration is corrected over a 24–48-hour period. Give fluids at 5 ml/kg only if the child is shocked and reassess regularly.

- Give high concentration oxygen and monitor arterial oxygen saturation (SpO_2)
- Establish venous access, but ideally give no fluid unless the patient is shocked or there is a prolonged delay to definitive care
- Fluids 5 ml/kg IV normal (0.9%) saline bolus only if the child is shocked
- Reassess, seek more skilled advice and repeat if necessary, this should be done in transit
- Further fluids should wait until hospital so that appropriate monitoring can be undertaken
- It is important to note how much fluid is given pre-hospital and hand this over on arrival

> **Insulin should be withheld until the patient is in hospital.**

Sickle cell crisis

Sickle cell disease is characterised by episodic clinical events called 'crises'. Vaso-occlusive crisis is the most common and occurs when abnormal red cells clog small vessels causing tissue ischaemia. The other crises are: hyper-haemolytic crisis; acute chest syndrome; sequestration crisis (severe anaemia and hypotension, resulting from pooling of blood in the spleen and liver); and aplastic crisis. Factors that precipitate or modulate the occurrence of sickle cell crises are not fully understood, but infections, hypoxia, dehydration, acidosis, stress and cold are believed to play some role.

Treatment

- Oxygen therapy
- Rehydration
- Parenteral morphine as required for pain
- Transfer to hospital

Cystic fibrosis

This is an inherited disorder, which primarily causes lung damage and malabsorption. Chronic complications are commonly respiratory and include chest infection. Patients are usually on a regime of antibiotics, inhaled medication and digestive enzyme supplements. The most likely presentation is an acute exacerbation of a chronic respiratory disease and patients will have their own protocol, or advice should be sought from their hospital team as they often have unusual pathogens with respiratory tract colonisation.

Treatment is as per the established protocol and/or for sepsis, i.e. oxygen, fluids and antibiotics as required.

Metabolic disorders

There are a large number of metabolic disorders that children may suffer from. These are also termed inborn errors of metabolism (IEM). They are frequently complex and should any child with an IEM present acutely unwell, urgent advice from their specialist team should be sought. The most likely presentations will be hypoglycaemia or metabolic acidosis and most, if not all, patients will have a care protocol for acute illness. Perform a blood glucose test in all patients with an IEM and acute illness. In the pre-hospital setting, actions likely to be required are correction of hypoglycaemia and treatment of shock (see Chapter 5). Transfer all patients with an IEM and acute illness to hospital for ongoing assessment unless it is clearly specified in care plans when it is safe not to do so.

10.3 Examples of equipment and troubleshooting

With advances in medicine, more children are now surviving with the assistance of equipment and appliances at home that would previously have been unheard of. Like all equipment, however, these machines and tubes can malfunction and the pre-hospital carer may now be called upon to assist in these emergencies.

Some of the commoner pieces of equipment and emergency solutions for mishaps or malfunctions are given in Table 10.1.

Table 10.1 Equipment: problems and solutions

Item	Function	Problem	Solution	Disposal and urgency
Tracheostomy tube	Provides patent airway when upper airway is obstructed	Blockage	• Confirm tube is correctly positioned • Remove the speech-cap from fenestrated tubes • Suction the tube to remove secretions (use the tube's obturator if suction is not available) • Remove the tracheostomy tube and replace • Ventilate to confirm correct position and patency	IMMEDIATE on scene Unless problem is easily resolved seek specialist advice and arrange admission
Home ventilator	Provides long-term ventilatory support	Equipment failure Loss of oxygen supply Loss of power	• Hand ventilate with bag–valve–mask and supplemental oxygen • Do not attempt to use machine unless trained	Immediate transfer to hospital
Ventriculoperitoneal (atrial) shunt	Drains CSF when not draining due to obstruction	Blockage – signs of raised intracranial pressure (irritability, abnormal cry, bulging fontanelles, etc.) Infection – signs of meningitis classically (may just have fever with no localising signs)		Transfer to hospital – if conscious level decreased give oxygen and support respiration Transfer to hospital – primary survey and management of ABCs
Central venous line	Venous access for: • drugs and blood taking • haemodialysis • parenteral nutrition	Bleeding – will also lead to risk of air embolism Line fracture Line infection	• Press on obvious bleeding round site • Check cap is tightened correctly • Place clamp proximally to any hole or perforation • Assess for sepsis	On scene Transport to hospital when bleeding is controlled Manage for air embolus if thought to have occurred: • cover with saline-soaked dressing • give 100% oxygen
Naso (oro) gastric tube	Access for enteral feeding, medications and fluids via a tube through the nose (mouth)	Displacement – pulled out	• Replace if trained	If not trained, transfer child to person who has been elected to replace tube as per child's care plan Monitor child's blood sugar if necessary to discontinue continuous tube feeds
		Possible dislodgement – coughing, history, etc.	• Check tube position if trained • Do not use if there are signs of respiratory distress	If not trained transfer as above Monitor child's blood sugar if necessary to discontinue continuous tube feeds

(*Continued*)

Table 10.1 (*Continued*)

Item	Function	Problem	Solution	Disposal and urgency
Gastrostomy – some are known as PEG (percutaneous enteral gastrostomy)	To provide feeding, etc. as above, directly into stomach through abdominal wall	Displacement	• Cover site with dressing	Immediate (but not emergency) transfer to suitable hospital
		Blockage	• Unblock as per carer's protocol if possible. Do not poke foreign objects down tube	Transfer to suitable hospital if unsuccessful
		Infection at site	• Clean site as per child's care plan	Contact child's specialist and arrange review Transfer to hospital, if child very unwell
Peritoneal dialysis catheter	Tube to allow fluid to run in and out of abdomen for dialysis	Peritonitis – cloudy dialysis fluid, abdominal pain May be other systemic symptoms of sepsis, including collapse	• Treat patient using ABC and primary survey. Give oxygen if required • Give 5 ml/kg aliquots of fluid if required to support circulation until stable. Do not overload • Follow care plan if available. If not, reapply cap/covering in as sterile a way as possible	Contact and transfer to hospital – urgency will be dictated by child's condition
		Disconnection/cap has come off Tube pulled out (rare)/ leaking	• Cover site with clean dressing	Contact and arrange transfer to hospital Contact hospital and arrange transfer
Urethral or suprapubic catheter	Drains urine from bladder (suprapubic through abdominal wall)	Tube pulled out	• Cover site if suprapubic	As for gastrostomy Contact hospital and arrange transfer
		Blocked catheter	• Unblock if trained, by flushing with saline using aseptic technique	If not resolved contact hospital and transfer urgently
		Infection at site (suprapubic)		As for gastrostomy

CHAPTER 11
Safeguarding children

Learning outcomes

After reading this chapter, you will be able to:
- Recognise abuse and neglect as a differential diagnosis
- Describe your approach to safeguarding children
- Describe the role of other agencies

11.1 Introduction

The United Nations Convention on the Rights of the Child 1989 provides a set of principles and standards to ensure that, among other things, children are protected. These apply to the practice of children's healthcare for all children and young people up to the age of 18 years. In the UK, unborn children are protected under the Children's Act 1989.

Article 3 provides that any decision or action affecting children either as individuals or as a group should be taken with 'their best interest' as the most important consideration

Article 9 holds that children have a right not to be separated from their parents or carers unless it is judged to be in their child's best interest

Article 12 obliges health professionals to seek a child's opinion before taking decisions that affect her or his future

Article 19 states that legislative, administrative, social and educational measures should be taken to protect children from all forms of physical and mental violence, injury and abuse (including sexual abuse) and negligent treatment

Article 37 states that no child shall be subjected to torture or other cruel, inhuman or degrading treatment or punishment

---

In 2012, World Health Organisation (WHO) data showed that 54 581 children died from intentional injuries globally; this is the equivalent of 150 children every day. In the UK TARN database, 10% of children under 2 years old were reported as being injured non-accidentally. Child abuse is a universal occurrence in all societies and in all parts of those societies.

This chapter focuses on generic principles associated with managing child abuse and neglect in the acute situation including recognition, urgent interventions and referral. Health professionals should seek guidance and legal details specific to their setting from national sources.

- Safeguarding is everyone's responsibility. If you have concerns that a child is being/has been abused you have a legal and professional obligation to act. The protection of the child takes priority over rules of confidentiality
- Abuse should always be considered as a potential differential diagnosis (it can often be rapidly excluded but if it is not thought about it will be missed)
- The pre-hospital picture is a vital part of the overall assessment and will guide decisions made by clinicians further down the care pathway. Accurate safeguarding decisions rely on a series of snap shots being assembled into an overall picture

---

Pre-Hospital Paediatric Life Support: A Practical Approach to Emergencies, Third Edition. Edited by Alan Charters, Hal Maxwell and Paul Reavley.
© 2017 John Wiley & Sons Ltd. Published 2017 by John Wiley & Sons Ltd.

Pre-hospital healthcare workers will come into contact with:

- Children who have been abused by adults or by other children
- Children who have abused other children
- Adults who were abused as children

There will also be contact with children who are present when assessing and treating other patients. It is possible that some of these children may have safeguarding requirements and pre-hospital healthcare workers must be vigilant for signs of abuse and neglect in all children present at the scene of the call, whether or not that child is the patient.

Present classifications are shown in Table 11.1.

Table 11.1 Classification of child abuse	
Neglect	The persistent failure to meet a child's basic physical and/or psychological needs, likely to result in the serious impairment of the child's health or development. Neglect may occur during pregnancy as a result of maternal substance abuse. Once a child is born, neglect may involve a parent or carer failing to: • provide adequate food, clothing and shelter (including exclusion from home or abandonment) • protect a child from physical and emotional harm or danger • ensure adequate supervision (including the use of inadequate care-givers) or • ensure access to appropriate medical care or treatment It may also include neglect of, or unresponsiveness to, a child's basic emotional needs
Physical abuse	A form of abuse that may involve hitting, shaking, throwing, poisoning, burning or scalding, drowning, suffocating or otherwise causing physical harm to a child. Physical harm may also be caused when a parent or carer fabricates the symptoms of, or deliberately induces, illness in a child
Sexual abuse	Involves forcing or enticing a child or young person to take part in sexual activities, not necessarily involving a high level of violence, whether or not the child is aware of what is happening. The activities may involve physical contact, including assault by penetration (e.g. rape or oral sex) or non-penetrative acts such as masturbation, kissing, rubbing and touching outside of clothing. They may also include non-contact activities, such as involving children in looking at, or in the production of, sexual images, watching sexual activities, encouraging children to behave in sexually inappropriate ways, or grooming a child in preparation for abuse (including via the internet). Sexual abuse is not solely perpetrated by adult males. Women can also commit acts of sexual abuse, as can other children
Emotional abuse	The persistent emotional maltreatment of a child such as to cause severe and persistent adverse effects on the child's emotional development. It may involve conveying to a child that they are worthless or unloved, inadequate or valued only insofar as they meet the needs of another person. It may include not giving the child opportunities to express their views, deliberately silencing them or 'making fun' of what they say or how they communicate. It may feature age or developmentally inappropriate expectations being imposed on children. These may include interactions that are beyond a child's developmental capability, as well as overprotection and limitation of exploration and learning, or preventing the child participating in normal social interaction. It may involve seeing or hearing the ill treatment of another. It may involve serious bullying (including cyber bullying), causing children frequently to feel frightened or in danger, or the exploitation or corruption of children. Some level of emotional abuse is involved in all types of maltreatment of a child, though it may occur alone

Susceptibility to abuse

The possibility of child ill treatment or abuse must be considered in the differential diagnosis of all children who have suffered injury. Child abuse/ill treatment occurs in all socioeconomic groups. However, the possible features of parenting known to be associated with child ill treatment or abuse include:

- Where the relationship between the parent and child does not appear loving and caring
- Where one or both parents have been abused themselves as children
- Parents who are young, single, unsupportive or substitutive
- Parents with learning difficulties
- Parents who have a poor or unstable relationship
- Situations where there is domestic violence and/or drug or alcohol dependence
- Parents who have mental illness or personality disorders

Factors in the child that make them vulnerable to abuse and ill treatment include:

- Prematurity
- Separation and impaired bonding in the neonatal period
- Physical or mental handicap
- Behavioural problems
- Difficult temperament or personality
- Soiling and wetting past developmental age
- Hyperactivity and attention deficit
- Screaming or crying interminably and inconsolably

11.2 Recognition of child abuse and neglect

As highlighted earlier, abuse should always be considered as a potential differential diagnosis. It can often be rapidly excluded but if it is not thought about, it will be missed. In emergency paediatrics consider the following key areas:

- Asphyxial event: suffocation, hanging
- Subdural haemorrhage
- Poisoning and other induced illness (e.g. septicaemia)
- Ruptured abdominal viscus
- Cervical spine injury
- Rib cage and long bone fractures
- Drowning
- Burns

Also, the following are presentations where you may have a higher index of suspicion:

Presentations of physical abuse

- Head injuries – fractures, intracranial injury. May present as an acute life-threatening event with breathing difficulty or apnoea. May present with raised intracranial pressure including symptoms or signs of poor feeding, vomiting, drowsiness or seizures
- Fractures of long bones – single fracture with multiple bruises, multiple fractures in different stages of healing, possibly with no bruises or soft tissue injury, or metaphyseal or epiphyseal injuries, often multiple
- Fractured ribs and spinal injuries
- Internal damage, e.g. rupture of bowel
- Burns and scalds – 'glove and stocking' appearance for scalds, implement imprints for contact burns
- Cold injury – hypothermia, frostbite
- Poisoning – drugs or household substances
- Suffocation
- Cuts and bruises – imprints of hands, sticks, whips, belts, bites, etc. may be present
- Bruising on non-prominent areas
- Bruising or injury in a non-mobile infant
- Collapsed infant

Presentations of sexual abuse

- Disclosure by child
- Disclosure by witness
- Suspicion by third party because of the behaviour of the child, especially changes in behaviour. These include insecurity; fear of men; sleep disorders; mood changes, tantrums and aggression at home; anxiety, despair, withdrawal and secretiveness; poor peer relationships; lying, stealing or arson; school failure; eating disorders like anorexia and compulsive overeating; running away and truancy; suicide attempts, self-poisoning, self-mutilation and abuse of drugs, solvents and alcohol; unexplained acquisition of money; sexualised behaviour such as drawings with a sexual content; knowledge of adult sexual behaviour shown in speech, play or drawing; apparent sexual approaches; and promiscuity
- Symptoms such as a sore bottom, vaginal discharge, bleeding per vagina in a pre-pubertal child, bleeding per rectum or inflamed penis which the care-giver believes is due to sexual abuse
- Symptoms as above and/or signs (e.g. unexplained perineal tear and/or bruising, torn hymen or perineal warts), but the doctor is the first person to suspect abuse

- Faecal soiling or relapse of enuresis
- Sexually transmitted disease
- Pregnancy but the girl refuses to name the putative father or even indicate the category, e.g. boyfriend, casual acquaintance
- Sexual intercourse with a child younger than 13 years is unlawful and therefore pregnancy in such a child means the child has been maltreated
- Female genital mutilation (FGM)

Presentations of neglect

- Severe and persistent infestations, such as scabies or head lice
- Severe dental disease
- A child's clothing or footwear is consistently inappropriate (e.g. for the weather or the child's size)
- A child is persistently smelly and dirty, especially if seen at times of the day when it is unlikely that they would have had an opportunity to become dirty or smelly (e.g. early morning)
- You repeatedly observe or hear reports of the home environment being of a poor standard of hygiene that affects a child's health
- The home environment is unsuitable for the child's stage of development and impacts on the child's safety or well-being. It may be difficult to distinguish between neglect and material poverty. However, care should be taken to balance recognition of the constraints on the parents' or carers' ability to meet their children's needs for food, clothing and shelter with an appreciation of how people in similar circumstances have been able to meet those needs
- Child abandonment
- Non-organic failure to thrive
- Repeated non-attendances at appointments that are necessary for the child's health and well-being
- Parents or carers fail to administer essential prescribed treatment for their child
- Parents or carers fail to seek medical advice for their child to the extent that the child's health and well-being is compromised
- Poor/inadequate supervision which may lead/has led to injury

---

It may be difficult to distinguish between deliberate neglect and material poverty. However, care should be taken to balance the recognition of constraints on the parents' or carers' ability to meet their children's need for food, clothing and shelter with an appreciation of how people in similar circumstances have been able to meet those needs. Equally some parents require exceptional support, such as those with learning difficulties or very young and isolated parents. Regardless of the presence of intent or otherwise, neglected children require safeguarding.

There are also some other pointers to be aware of during your history taking and examination:

- There is delay in seeking medical help or medical help is not sought at all
- The story of the 'accident' is vague, is lacking in detail and may vary with each telling and from person to person. Innocent accidents tend to have vivid accounts that ring true
- The account of the accident is not compatible with the injury observed or is inconsistent between parents and carers
- The injury is not compatible with the child's level of development or of the level of development of another child alleged to have caused the injury
- The parents' affect is abnormal. Note anything that appears abnormal to you in this regard
- The parents' behaviour gives cause for concern. They may become hostile, rebut accusations that have not been made or leave before the consultant arrives
- The child's appearance and his interaction with his parents are abnormal. He may look sad, withdrawn or frightened. There may be visible evidence of failure to thrive. Full-blown frozen watchfulness is a late stage and results from repetitive physical and emotional abuse over a period of time

---

Other safeguarding concerns

- Alcohol or drug use
- Deliberate self-harm
- High-risk sexual behaviour

11.3 Assessment

The assessment of all children should follow the standard < C > ABCDE and full medical assessment approach.

Consent for examination is mandatory in all cases unless a serious life-threatening injury is suspected. This needs to be given by an adult with parental responsibility or the child if competent. Social care may need to get a court order if appropriate consent is not available or refused. This is also an aspect that will be subject to national laws, policies and procedures and you should familiarise yourself with those relevant to your practice using national guidance.

Details of medical assessment: history

A full history should be taken as in any medical assessment. There are some specific issues to consider if child abuse or neglect is on your list of differential diagnoses:

- Full details of the history of the incident(s) should be obtained from the child and the care-givers. If social workers and police officers have previously talked to the child, then taking this history from them may be appropriate, especially for alleged sexual offences. Frequent repetition of the details can be very disturbing to the child and can jeopardise evidence
- In history related to the gastrointestinal tract remember to ask about soiling, constipation, rectal pain and rectal bleeding
- In history related to the urogenital system remember to ask about wetting, vaginal bleeding, vaginal discharge and, when appropriate, menarche, cycle, sanitary protection and previous sexual intercourse
- Personal history must start with the mother's pregnancy, birth, the neonatal period and subsequent developmental milestones. Then details of immunisations, drug history (including alcohol and street drugs) and allergies are obtained
- Enquiries are made about previous illnesses and injuries, with dates of attendance at hospital or at the surgery of the family doctor. Past records should be obtained and relevant information should be extracted
- The traditional family history should include details of the natural parents, all co-habitees and any other people who regularly care for the child, e.g. relatives and childminders
- Parental illness should be discussed, particularly psychiatric illness
- The possibility of domestic abuse should be explored
- Then the names, ages and medical histories of all siblings and half-siblings are obtained
- Familial illnesses that are particularly important are inherited skin, musculoskeletal or blood disorders
- Enquire if the family has any community paediatric or social work input and the name of a community paediatrician, named social worker or key worker

Remember to remain objective and show professional sensitivity. Document who is present and their relationship to the child. Use open questions and avoid leading questions. Full contemporaneous notes are essential at all stages of a safeguarding process.

Additional information should be sought from social care or emergency duty teams out of hours. They will be able to inform you if the child or other children in the family are subject to current or previous safeguarding plans and if they have named key workers.

Examination

Ensure an appropriate chaperone is present. The general examination starts while the history is being taken. During that time the pre-hospital care provider observes the affect of the child, the relationships between the child, mother, father and others present and any behavioural problems. If the child is reluctant to be examined, then playing with toys or a stethoscope often breaks the ice. No child should be examined against his or her will as this constitutes an assault.

General assessment

- Comment on the pre-hospital environment including other family members and non-family present
- Full head to toe examination
- Comment on general level of hygiene, clothing, etc.
- Document any injuries on pre-hospital records
- Comment on developmental level and interaction with carers

If possible a full head to toe assessment should be performed at some point in the care pathway when abuse or neglect is suspected. If this is not possible because of the environment or pre-hospital dynamics then this should occur in hospital. Document the limitations of the examination and ensure that it is handed over to receiving clinicians.

Sexual abuse examination

- Such an examination should be always undertaken by a doctor with the necessary competences
- The examination should never be attempted by pre-hospital practitioners unless serious injury that requires immediate treatment is evident
- If there has been an acute assault then forensic examination will be needed – often this is as a joint examination with the paediatrician and forensic medical examiner

11.4 Initial management

Medical treatment is the priority if the child has serious or life-, limb- or sight-threatening injuries. At the end of the medical assessment the diagnosis may be clear. More often, there is a differential diagnosis that includes abuse.

For paediatric trauma, ask the following questions:

- Does the story of the mechanism fit with the injury pattern seen? (e.g. a 'fall down the stairs' with bruising on the abdomen)
- Do the injuries fit with what is reasonable for this child's developmental age? (e.g. a 1-month-old baby who 'rolled off the bed')
- Could the parents or carers have done anything in advance to prevent the accident happening? (e.g. a burn injury in an unsupervised toddler)
- Could the parents or carers have done anything after the accident to improve medical care? (e.g. an injury which has not had prompt care)

When the diagnosis or differential diagnosis is one of child abuse then the decisions to be made on management are the following:

- Does the child need hospital assessment for treatment of the injuries?
- Will the child be safe if returned home?
- If the child needs protection from an abuser who is in his or her own home, how can this be done?
- What support/protection is needed for the rest of the family, including siblings? If one child is at risk, then others in the home may also be assumed to be at risk

11.5 What to do if there are safeguarding concerns

The first priority is to meet the child's immediate health needs and provide emergency treatment for injury or illness as you normally would for any other patient. If hospital assessment is required, the child should be transported when clinically appropriate, but carefully note the scene and social factors as discussed previously. These may be vital at a later point. On arrival at hospital ensure that you have handed over your safeguarding concerns to the receiving clinician. In these circumstances, where hospital assessment is clearly required regardless of safeguarding concerns, the hospital will be able to communicate with all necessary other agencies.

Always complete a 'Cause for concern' form or equivalent safeguarding notification. Even if this will be done again in hospital, this will add to the overall picture.

The pre-hospital environment can be a difficult place to assess the need for safeguarding. If neglect or abuse cannot be excluded to the satisfaction of the clinician then get help and advice from:

- Community paediatrics
- Social workers
- Police
- Emergency department

If, at any time there is a perceived immediate risk to the child, call the police at once.

Where there are concerns of child abuse and neglect, discussion takes place among the various agencies. This is done in order to balance the probabilities of abuse having occurred and to establish on-going risk. Approaches to this will vary from country to country, but in all cases should include a decision about whether it may be necessary to arrange for the child to be taken to a place of safety or if they can safely remain in their current environment.

If abuse and neglect are likely then a multi-agency assessment involving social care, health and the police will be required. As a separate, parallel process, the police will consider whether criminal investigation is appropriate or necessary; in many cases a full criminal investigation will not take place. The approach to this will vary according to national laws, policies and procedures.

All child protection work is based on cooperation between families, social workers, police officers, healthcare workers and educationalists. This multi-agency approach is to ensure that all aspects of the care of the family are considered when decisions are being made. Certain decisions in management must be made by a professional, e.g. only a doctor can decide on the treatment required for a fracture and only a police officer can decide the charge that is appropriate for the alleged offence. However, whenever possible, unilateral decisions are avoided in the best interests of the child and the family.

Healthcare workers may be concerned about sharing information with other professionals because of the ethical consideration of confidentiality. In the UK, the General Medical Council (2012) gives the following advice.

Ask for consent to share information unless there is a compelling reason for not doing so. Information can be shared without consent if it is justified in the public interest or required by law. Do not delay disclosing information to obtain consent if that might put children or young people at risk of significant harm.

Advice on consent will vary from country to country and you should be aware of your own national guidance and advice.

11.6 Medicolegal aspects

Healthcare professionals must be familiar with the medicolegal aspects of their work. These may vary according to the jurisdiction where the clinician practices. They will in most cases cover the following:

- Court orders to enable:
  - Emergency protection
  - Child assessment
  - Residence
  - Police protection
- Consent to examination

In some cases where there is involvement of either a criminal or family court, healthcare professionals may be required to write statements and/or present evidence.

Statements

The purpose of a statement is to provide the court with an informative and relevant factual account of the medical assessment of the child rather than the opinion of the individual writing it. The statement will give details of the persons involved, the observations and the findings. Information given by another person should not be included unless this has been requested. In many areas, the prosecutors wish statements to record all information, although hearsay may be excluded before presentation to the court.

A statement is a professional document. It should be well written in clear, readily understandable language. Technical terms should be avoided or, if used, should be followed immediately by appropriate lay terms. Most statements will be for the prosecution and a printed statement form will be provided. The standard sequence of writing a statement is shown in the following box.

Statements must be completed in the format required by the legal authorities. Clinicians should keep copies of statements submitted in keeping with data protection guidance.

Suggested sequence for writing statements

- Full name with surname in capitals
- Qualifications
- Occupation
- Name of child
- Date, time and place of contact with the child
- Name/s of persons present
- Details of the relevant history
- Details of examination
- Treatment given
- Opinion on findings (if acting as an expert witness)
- Time at which contact with the child ended
- Date the report is made

Each page of the statement must be signed at the bottom and the final page must be signed on the line below the completion of the writing. Any alterations must be initialled. Always keep a copy of the statement.

Presentation of evidence

Dress in a professional manner. Arrive early in court. Take along all notes relevant to the case. Review these on the day before the court proceedings, as well as your report. With permission from the magistrate or judge, you may refer to contemporaneous notes. However, thorough preparation helps to put the whole picture of the incident into the forefront of your mind so that you can find the appropriate notes more quickly.

When giving evidence stay calm even when challenged. Do not be persuaded to answer questions that are outside your knowledge or experience. Opinion on cause and effect is purely the domain of the expert witness.

11.7 Summary

- Safeguarding is everyone's responsibility
- If you have concerns that a child is being/has been abused you have an obligation to refer
- Abuse should always be considered as a potential differential diagnosis – it can often be rapidly excluded, but if it is not thought about it will be missed

CHAPTER 12
Pain management in children

Learning outcomes

After reading this chapter, you will be able to:
- Recognise and quantify pain in children
- Describe your approach to treating pain
- Describe the common analgesic drugs and routes of administration

---

12.1 Introduction

Excellent pain control is an essential and basic standard in the management of injured children. Practitioners should aim to control pain as soon as possible. Analgesia will reduce tachycardia and bleeding, manage distress and result in a calmer, more cooperative child. The essential steps in achieving this are firstly recognition – pain should be anticipated at all times and we must be vigilant for all signs. Secondly, a comprehensive knowledge of the agents and routes available to the pre-hospital practitioner is required. Full dosing information can be found in the Appendix. This information does not replace local guideline and policy, all drug doses should be checked against the current *British National Formulary for Children* (BNFc).

12.2 Assessment

All children require documented pain scores at regular intervals, both pre and post analgesia. The preference is that children self-report pain where possible. Older children may be able to give a pain score when asked but for younger children the practitioner will need to make an objective assessment using an appropriate and validated pain assessment tool combining physiological and behavioural responses to pain. There are many such tools, most of which are appropriate for the post-operative or peri-procedural setting, although none are yet validated in the pre-hospital setting. Two tools appropriate for the acute pain or emergency department setting are the Alder Hey Triage Pain Scale (Table 12.1), suitable for children of all ages,

Table 12.1 The Alder Hey Triage Pain Scale: reference scoring chart

Response	Score 0	Score 1	Score 2
Cry/voice	No complaint/cry	Consolable	Inconsolable
	Normal conversation	Not talking negative	Complaining of pain
Facial expression	Normal	Short grimace <50% time	Long grimace >50% time
Posture	Normal	Touching/rubbing/sparing	Defensive/tense
Movement	Normal	Reduced or restless	Immobile or thrashing
Colour	Normal	Pale	Very pale/'green'

Pre-Hospital Paediatric Life Support: A Practical Approach to Emergencies, Third Edition. Edited by Alan Charters, Hal Maxwell and Paul Reavley
© 2017 John Wiley & Sons Ltd. Published 2017 by John Wiley & Sons Ltd.

and the Colour Pain Scale (Figure 12.1). Other commonly used tools include the Faces Scale and Pain Ladder (Figure 12.2), the Wong Baker FACES® Pain Rating Scale (Figure 12.3) and the FLACC Behavioural Pain Assessment Scale (Table 12.2). Practitioners must remember that the behavioural response to pain is culturally variable and the absence of a behavioural response does not indicate an absence of pain. Equally, we must never perceive the patient's pain to be less than they express.

Guidance notes for the use of the Alder Hey score can be found in Section 12.3.

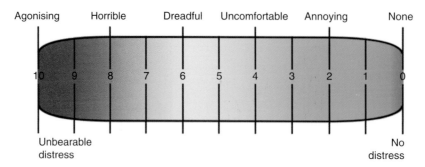

Figure 12.1 Colour Pain Scale

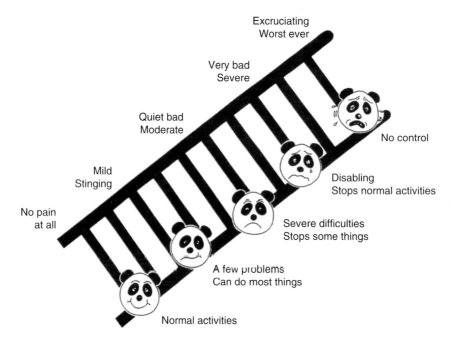

Figure 12.2 Faces Scale and Pain Ladder

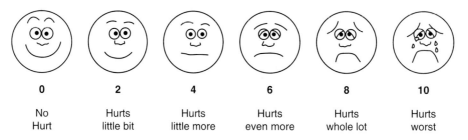

Figure 12.3 Wong Baker FACES® Pain Rating Scale. Source: Wong-Baker FACES Foundation (2015). Wong Baker FACES® Pain Rating Scale. Retrieved Jan 2017. Reproduced with permission of Wong-Baker FACES Foundation http://www.WongBakerFACES.org

Table 12.2 FLACC scale

Criteria	Score 0	Score 1	Score 2
Face	No particular expression or smile	Occasional grimace or frown, withdrawn, uninterested	Frequent to constant quivering chin, clenched jaw
Legs	Normal position or relaxed	Uneasy, restless, tense	Kicking, or legs drawn up
Activity	Lying quietly, normal position, moves easily	Squirming, shifting, back and forth, tense	Arched, rigid or jerking
Cry	No cry (awake or asleep)	Moans or whimpers; occasional complaint	Crying steadily, screams or sobs, frequent complaints
Consolability	Content, relaxed	Reassured by occasional touching, hugging or being talked to, distractible	Difficult to console or comfort

12.3 Analgesia

Oral analgesia

Where possible, all children should receive oral analgesia when in pain even if parenteral routes have been used. Such analgesia is extremely effective and if given early will establish some longer acting analgesia once parenteral agents are wearing off and the child is packaged. Oral analgesics include paracetamol, ibuprofen and opioids.

Codeine is now contraindicated in all children less than 12 years of age and in children 12–18 years of age who are post tonsillectomy or adenoidectomy with a history of sleep apnoea. Alternatives to codeine are dihydrocodeine, oral morphine solution and tramadol (see Table 12.3).

Rectal analgesia

This is a useful route in distressed or vomiting infants. Both paracetamol and diclofenac can be administered via the rectal route.

Intravenous analgesia

Titrated intravenous opiates remain the gold standard for the control of severe pain. However, intravenous access can be difficult to achieve and can cause distress for the child. It can also be a cause of unacceptable scene delay. For most children pain will be controlled by alternative routes. Analgesics suitable for intravenous administration include paracetamol, morphine, fentanyl and ketamine (see Table 12.3).

Intraosseus analgesia

If the intraosseus route is available it can be used for all intravenous analgesic drugs at the same dose.

Intramuscular analgesia

Intramuscular ketamine is a rapid and effective route to deliver good pain control. It is particularly useful in burns where the patient is both very distressed and is difficult to cannulate. Whilst there are analgesic, sedative and anaesthetic doses quoted, the reality is that the distinction can be difficult to achieve. Practically, any ketamine use in children will produce some altered consciousness, therefore monitoring, equipment and safety requirements should be those used for procedural sedation.

In the presence of shock the intramuscular route is far less effective. In particular, there is no role for intramuscular opiates in the analgesic strategy.

Intranasal analgesia

This is a particularly useful route to achieve effective and rapid analgesia. Ketamine, fentanyl and diamorphine are all well absorbed through the nasal mucosa. Diamorphine is commonly used in UK emergency departments to relieve initial burn and fracture pain prior to gaining intravenous access. Initially piloted in 1998 there have been no reported incidents of significant adverse effects and it is extremely well tolerated. The drugs need to be in a low volume, and volumes above 0.4 ml should be divided between nostrils. At above 0.4 ml efficacy may be lost as more of the drug is swallowed rather than absorbed via the mucosa. The drugs should be administered using a 1 ml syringe and a mucosal atomiser device (MAD) or by delivery systems now available in the UK. Fentanyl is a suitable alternative and is widely used where diamorphine is not available, such as in Australia. Doses for intranasal drugs are detailed in Table 12.4.

Inhaled analgesia

Older children, probably around school age and above, will be able to use inhaled agents such as nitrous oxide and oxygen mix. This will provide temporary but not definitive pain relief. The child is likely to be more cooperative once some analgesia/sedation secondary to the nitrous oxide is achieved. This may allow the practitioner to gain intravenous access, dress or splint the injury and provide further pain relief. Do not use nitrous oxide in the presence of a pneumothorax, as the nitrous oxide will diffuse into the cavity and cause it to expand.

Peripheral nerve blocks

There is limited utility for pre-hospital nerve blocks in children. However, they can be of use, particularly in femoral bone fractures, for which femoral nerve blocks or fascia iliaca compartment blocks can provide excellent pain control. It is advisable to practice ultrasound guided rather than blind techniques where applicable and practitioners must be trained and experienced in any peripheral nerve block they wish to use.

Non-pharmacological analgesia

Never underestimate the powers of the 'magic bandage'. Children in pain need reassurance and comfort – be nice. Dressing wounds will reduce pain, in particular burns, which should be dressed with cling film to prevent stimulation from air movement over the affected area. Commercial cooling dressings are also available for burn management. Covering wounds will also reduce the psychological impact of the appearance, helping to calm the patient.

Extremity wounds should be immobilised and elevated or placed in a sling. Carrying an appropriate selection of splint devices such as malleable, vacuum and traction splints will enable the immobilisation of most wounds and fractures. This is particularly important during extraction and transfer as there is likely to be some movement. Remember to check neurovascular status before and regularly after placing a limb in splintage.

Sucrose/dextrose

Oral sweet solutions can be used as a mild analgesic in infants. It is most effective in neonates but has been shown to have some effect, both analgesic and calming up to the age of 18 months.

Indications

Sucrose should only be used for the reduction of brief, mild, procedural pain, for example cannula insertion and for short-term management of distress when other comfort measures have failed. The analgesic action lasts for a few minutes only, therefore sucrose is not appropriate for the management of continuing pain or distress. If the pain is more than mild, sucrose should not be used in place of other appropriate analgesia.

In infants and younger children the following measures may also help in reducing distress:

- Breastfeeding or non-nutritive sucking using a dummy if is a normal part of the infant's care, and if the infant is able to suck
- Full or partial swaddling
- Reduction in noxious stimuli and overstimulation, e.g. noise and lighting
- Holding and cuddling with a parent or carer
- Support infants over 6 months old in the upright position where possible
- Distraction for older infants, e.g. toys, music, etc.

Table 12.3 Drug doses for analgesia

Drug	Route*	Dose	Cautions
Paracetamol	Oral Rectal Intravenous	15 mg/kg (max. 1 g) QDS 15 mg/kg (max. 1 g) QDS Over 10 kg: 15 mg/kg (max. 1 g) QDS Under 10 kg: 7.5 mg/kg QDS (max. 30 mg/kg/day)	Always check if paracetamol has been administered by carers
Ibuprofen	Oral only	5 mg/kg (max. 400 mg) TDS	May exacerbate asthma. Avoid in renal disease, gastric ulceration and bleeding disorders
Diclofenac	Oral Rectal	1 mg/kg (max. 50 mg) TDS 1 mg/kg (max. 50 mg) TDS	May exacerbate asthma. Avoid in renal disease, gastric ulceration and bleeding disorders
Codeine	Oral only	1 mg/kg (max. 60 mg) QDS	Contraindications below[†]
Tramadol	Oral Intravenous	1 mg/kg (max. 50 mg) QDS 1 mg/kg (max. 50 mg) QDS	Serotonergic side effects
Oramorph	Oral only	1–3 months: 50–100 mcg/kg 4-hourly 3–6 months: 100–150 mcg/kg 4-hourly 6–12 months: 100–200 mcg/kg 4-hourly >1 year: 200–300 mcg/kg 4-hourly	Respiratory and CNS depression. Nausea and vomiting
Sucrose 24–33% Dextrose 25–50% See notes below	Oral onto tongue only	0–1 month 1 ml 1–18 months 1–2 ml Given in small incremental doses during procedure	Sucrose/fructose intolerance Glucose galactose malabsorption
Morphine	Intravenous only	50 mcg/kg boluses up to 200 mcg/kg titrated to pain	Respiratory and CNS depression. Nausea and vomiting
Fentanyl	Intravenous Intranasal	0.25 mcg/kg in boluses up to 1 mcg/kg titrated to pain 1 mcg/kg atomised into nostril(s)	Respiratory and CNS depression. Nausea and vomiting If >0.4 ml, divide between nostrils
Diamorphine	Intranasal	See Table 12.5	Respiratory and CNS depression. Nausea and vomiting
Ketamine (sedation and analgesia)	Intravenous Intramuscular Intranasal	0.25–0.5 mg/kg 2–4 mg/kg 3 mg/kg	Dysphoria Consider small dose of benzodiazepine

* Intravenous doses apply to intraosseus route also.

† Codeine is now contraindicated in all children less than 12 years of age and in children aged 12–18 years of age who are post tonsillectomy or adenoidectomy with a history of sleep apnoea. Alternatives to codeine are dihydrocodeine, oral morphine solution and tramadol.

CNS, central nervous system; QDS, four times a day; TDS, three times a day.

How to give oral sucrose
* Draw up the amount of sucrose/dextrose to be given orally (Table 12.3)
* Give approximately one-quarter of the total amount of sucrose 2 minutes prior to the start of the procedure. Doses are to be placed directly onto the tongue
* Offer a dummy if this is a normal part of the infant's care, this will be calming
* Give the rest of the dose incrementally throughout the procedure
* The analgesic effect lasts 5–8 minutes. If ineffective or pain is ongoing, give stronger and longer acting analgesia

Table 12.4 Intranasal diamorphine dosing table (using 10 mg vial of diamorphine)

Weight/kg	Volume saline added/ml	Notes
15	1.3	1. Estimate weight or weigh to nearest 5 kg
20	1.0	2. Add weight-specific volume of 0.9% sodium chloride
25	0.8	3. Draw up 0.2 ml of the solution
30	0.7	4. Once drawn up administer into nostril using a mucosal atomiser device. This will deliver 0.1 mg/kg of diamorphine
35	0.6	
40	0.5	
50	0.4	
60	0.3	

Wilson JA, Kendall JM, Cornelius P. Intranasal diamorphine for paediatric analgesia: assessment of safety and efficacy. *J Accid Emerg Med* 1997 Mar;14(2):70–2.

12.4 Explanatory notes for the Alder Hey Triage Pain Scale

Cry/voice

Score 0   Child is not crying and, although may be quiet, is vocalising appropriately with carer or taking notice of surroundings

Score 1   Child is crying but consolable/distractible or is excessively quiet and responding negatively to carer. On direct questioning says it is painful

Score 2   Child is inconsolable, crying and/or persistently complaining about pain

Facial expression

Score 0   Normal expression and affect

Score 1   Some transient expressions that suggest pain/distress are witnessed but less than 50% of time

Score 2   Persistent facial expressions suggesting pain/distress more than 50% of time

Grimace: open mouth, lips pulled back at corners, furrowed forehead and/or between eyebrows, eyes closed, wrinkled at corners.

Posture

This relates to the child's behaviour to the affected body area.

Score 0   Normal

Score 1   Exhibiting increased awareness of affected area, e.g. by touching, rubbing, pointing, sparing or limping

Score 2   Affected area is held tense and defended so that touching it is deterred; non-weight-bearing

Movement

This relates to how the child moves the whole body.

Score 0   Normal
Score 1   Movement is reduced or child is noted to be restless/uncomfortable
Score 2   Movement is abnormal, either very still/rigid or writhing in agony/shaking

Colour

Score 0   Normal
Score 1   Pale
Score 2   Very pale 'green', the colour that can sometimes be seen with nausea or fainting – extreme pallor

CHAPTER 13
Paediatric triage

Learning outcomes

After reading this chapter, you will be able to:
• Understand the importance of pre-hospital triage
• Describe a triage system

13.1 Introduction

Definition

Triage is the process of sorting multiple patients into priorities for treatment.

Triage is commonly thought to be relevant only in the circumstances of major incidents and trauma but it is a process undertaken whenever the number or type of potential casualties exceed immediate resources. Thus a single paramedic responding to two ill children in the same house will need to conduct a rapid triage exercise to establish both which of the children he or she needs to deal with first and to decide what additional resources are needed.

It is vital to observe that triage is a dynamic process that must be repeated at every link of the evacuation chain. The priority for action may change if there is any clinical change in the child.

Triage requires that each child presenting with potentially serious illness or injury is assigned a clinical priority. As such the triage process can be seen to be an extension of the process of recognition of the seriously ill or injured child.

Triage assigns treatment priorities as below:

• Priority 1 (red) – requires immediate life-saving treatment
• Priority 2 (yellow) – requires urgent definitive treatment within 2–4 hours
• Priority 3 (green) – those whose treatment can be delayed for >4 hours

Importantly, in a multiple casualty situation the rescuer must not attempt to predict how the patient's condition may change. This will inevitably lead to over-triage, and a disproportionate number of priority 1 and priority 2 casualties.

It is also important that when conducting triage, decisions are made quickly, safely and reproducibly, whether the person conducting the triage assessment is a first aider or consultant paediatrician.

Pre-Hospital Paediatric Life Support: A Practical Approach to Emergencies, Third Edition. Edited by Alan Charters, Hal Maxwell and Paul Reavley.
© 2017 John Wiley & Sons Ltd. Published 2017 by John Wiley & Sons Ltd.

13.2 Seriously injured children

A recent study looking back over 30 years has revealed that major incidents occur in the UK on average three or four times per year, and up to 11 times per year. The evidence confirms that the majority of major incidents do involve a proportion of children and a number of incidents predominantly or exclusively involve children.

There are two identifiable approaches to managing an incident that involves injured children. Some would argue that *all* children should be given the highest treatment priority (priority 1, immediate). After all, every child is dependent to some degree. While this approach can be understood, the danger is that the limited hospital paediatric resources will be diluted, and key personnel will be unavailable to treat the child in genuine urgent need. Additionally, it is difficult to argue rationally why a child should be treated before a more seriously injured adult. The strategy also becomes corrupt when dealing with incidents involving only children, for example a school bus in a road traffic collision. Triaging all patients into the highest priority could conceal the most seriously injured child and delay life-saving treatment.

The alternative approach is to prioritise children according to their clinical need, in parallel with adults who are ill or have been injured.

Methods of triage

Triage following injury can be anatomical, physiological or a mixture of the two. Anatomical methods rely on assigning a priority according to the injuries that are evident on physical examination. This has a number of inherent problems:

- The patient must be undressed, which is both time consuming and impractical outside hospital
- Triage will be inconsistent between observers, depending on their clinical experience
- Some life-threatening conditions will be missed by clinical examination alone – e.g. haemoperitoneum is only detected in 35% of cases by examination of the abdomen

Physiological methods assess the consequences of injury. They have been shown to be simple, safe, rapid and reproducible between observers. The principal disadvantages of these methods are:

- The majority are based on adult physiological parameters leading to over-triage of children
- In the early period following injury, there will be physiological compensation, leading to under-triage

Mixed methods allow clinical experience to influence the physiological triage priority, but this will introduce inconsistency when there are observers with a range of clinical experience.

Physiological methods of triage are preferred outside of hospital. Initial triage is done using a simple scheme known as *triage sieve*. Once the child is in a more secure environment, e.g. a hospital emergency department, or in the case of a major incident, a casualty clearing station, a more detailed assessment is undertaken using the *triage sort*. This refines the priority by adding more clinical and physiological information, including systolic blood pressure and Glasgow Coma Scale score.

Triage sieve

A widely used physiological triage system in the UK (both civilian and military) and Australia is the *triage sieve*. The priority categories correlate directly with the commonly used T1, T2 and T3 categories. This uses a simple algorithm to assess mobility, followed by a rapid assessment of <C>ABC. Specifically, there is a need to count the respiratory rate and the pulse or capillary refill time (Figure 13.1).

Any child that has been treated for catastrophic haemorrhage is a priority 1.

Any child who is trapped and cannot therefore be appropriately or fully assessed is likewise a priority 1 *at this point in time*.

The *triage sieve,* however, uses adult physiological parameters and for this reason the system has been modified to produce the paediatric triage tape (Figure 13.2).

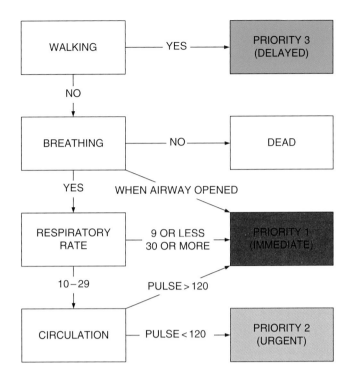

Figure 13.1 Paediatric triage sieve

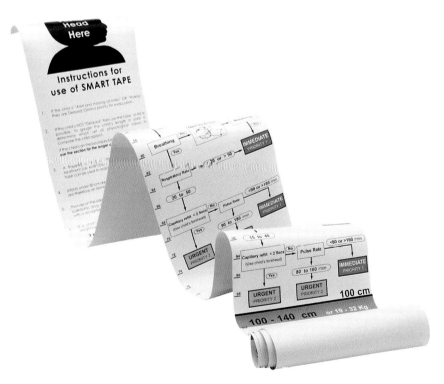

Figure 13.2 Paediatric triage tape. Reproduced with permission of TSG Associates LLP (England) www.smartmci.com

The length of a child is proportional to his or her weight and age. This principle is employed through various paediatric emergency tapes such as the Sandell and Broselow tapes. These relate a child's length to the correct dose of resuscitation drugs and therapies, and other important medications and equipment. In the same way, the length of a child can be related to the normal physiological parameters for that age. This is the foundation of the paediatric triage tape. The tape is a series of triage sieve algorithms with respiratory and pulse rates corrected for the length (and age and weight) of the child.

Mobility assessment is also necessarily different, with an infant being assessed as 'mobile' if he or she is moving all limbs spontaneously.

Additionally, the capillary refill time (CRT) is only used to screen for a normal circulation. If the CRT is delayed, a pulse must still be taken. Children cool quickly, and CRT may be falsely delayed in the cold. It is recommended that the forehead be used to take the CRT in children. The limited experimental evidence on CRT shows that the only normal distribution of values is when it is performed on the forehead or the sternum (but the sternum requires exposing pre-hospital). The nail bed and the heel produce inconsistent results.

When the tape cannot be used in a trapped child, the child is automatically assigned priority 1. Once extrication is complete, the triage priority is reassessed using the tape alongside the child.

Triage for illness

In most out of hospital care, ill children will present singly and as such triage to determine treatment priorities is not required.

The decision to be made will be the severity of the illness and therefore the urgency needed in transfer of the child to definitive care.

Examples of children needing urgent transfer are those with:

- Any cessation or threat to the vital (ABC) functions, e.g. the presence of an insecure airway, inspiratory or expiratory stridor, absent or inadequate breathing, shock
- Non-blanching petechial rash
- Severe pain
- Change in the level of consciousness
- New-onset convulsions
- Illness not responding to initial resuscitation interventions

CHAPTER 14
Human factors

Learning outcomes

After reading this chapter, you will be able to:
• Describe how human factors affect the performance of individuals and teams in the healthcare environment

14.1 Introduction

The emphasis on the management of paediatric emergency care has traditionally concentrated on knowledge of the treatment process, for example when to give a specific intervention, drug or aliquot of fluid. An often overlooked element is how in these high-pressure situations individuals from a variety of different professional and specialty backgrounds come together to form an effective team that minimises errors and works actively to prevent adverse events.

This chapter provides a brief introduction to some of the human factors that can affect the performance of individuals and teams in the healthcare environment. Human factors, also referred to as ergonomics, is an established scientific discipline and clinical human factors has been described as:

> Enhancing clinical performance through an understanding of the effects of teamwork, tasks, equipment, workspace, culture and organisation on human behaviour and abilities and application of that knowledge in clinical settings. (Catchpole, 2010)

14.2 Extent of healthcare error

In 2000 an influential report entitled *To Err is Human: Building a Safer Health System* (Catchpole, 2010) suggested that across the USA somewhere between 44 000 and 98 000 deaths each year could be attributed to medical error. A pilot study in the UK demonstrated that approximately one in 10 patients admitted to healthcare experienced an adverse event.

Healthcare has been able to learn from a number of other high-risk industries including the nuclear, petrochemical, space exploration, military and aviation industries about how team issues have been managed. These lessons have been slowly adopted and translated to healthcare.

Specialist working groups and national bodies have been instrumental in promoting awareness of the importance of human factors in healthcare. They aim to raise awareness and promote the principles and practices of human factors, identify current human factor activity, capability and barriers, and create conditions to support human factors being embedded at a local level. One such example of this is the Human Factors Clinical Working Group and the National Quality Board's concordat statement on human factors.

Pre-Hospital Paediatric Life Support: A Practical Approach to Emergencies, Third Edition. Edited by Alan Charters, Hal Maxwell and Paul Reavley.
© 2017 John Wiley & Sons Ltd. Published 2017 by John Wiley & Sons Ltd.

14.3 Causes of healthcare error

Consider this example of an adverse event:

A child needs to receive an infusion of a particular drug. An error occurs and the child receives an incorrect drug. What are the potential causes of this situation?

Potential causes of our example drug error	
Prescription error	Wrong drug prescribed
Preparation error	Correct drug prescribed but misread
Preparation error	Contents mislabelled during manufacture
Drawing up error	Incorrect drug selected
Administration error	Patient ID mix-up, drug given to wrong patient

Q. What one thing links all of these errors?
A. The humans involved – these are all examples of human errors.

Humans make mistakes. No amount of checks and procedures will mitigate this fact. In fact the only way to completely remove human error is to remove all the humans involved. It is vital therefore that we look to work in a way that, wherever possible, minimises the occurrence of mistakes and ensures that when they do occur the method minimises the chance of the error resulting in an adverse event.

14.4 Human error

It has been suggested that these human errors can be further categorised into: (i) those that occur at the sharp end of care by the treating team and individuals; and (ii) those that occur at the blunt or organisational level, typically through policies, procedures, staffing and culture. These errors can be further subdivided (Table 14.1).

Table 14.1 Types of errors		Explanation	Example
Sharp errors that occur with the team/individuals treating the patient	Mistake	Lack or misapplication of knowledge	Not knowing the correct drug to prescribe
	Slip or lapse	Skills-based mistake	Knowing the correct drug but writing another one
	Violation	Deliberate action that may be routine or exceptional	Not attempting to get a drug second checked as there are no staff available
Blunt/organisational errors		Policies, procedures, infrastructure and building layout that has errors embedded	Different drugs used by different specialities and departments for same condition

It is typically found that the latent/organisational issues often coexist with the sharp errors; in fact it is rare for an isolated error to occur – often there is a chain of events that results in the adverse event. The 'Swiss cheese' model demonstrates how apparently random, unconnected events and organisational decisions can all make errors more likely (Figure 14.1). Conversely, a standardised system with good defences can capture these errors and prevent adverse events.

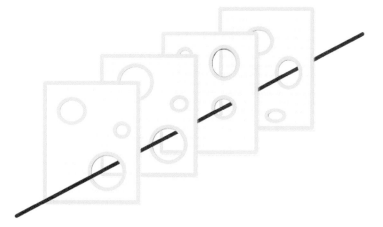

Figure 14.1 The 'Swiss cheese' model

Each of the slices of Swiss cheese represents barriers that, under ideal circumstances, would prevent or detect the error. The holes represent weaknesses in these barriers; if the holes align the error passes through undetected.

Reconsider the example of drug error using the Swiss cheese model. The first slice is the doctor writing the prescription, the second slice is the organisation's drug policy, the third is the nurse who draws up the drug and the fourth is the nurse who second checks the drug.

Now consider the following: What if the doctor is inexperienced and not familiar with that area or drugs used? – their slice of cheese has larger holes. What if the organisation has failed to develop a robust drug policy that is fit for purpose? – this second slice is considerably weakened or may even be removed completely. What if the paramedic is new to the unit and unfamiliar with unit practice? – their slice has also got larger holes. What if this area is always short of staff so that other staff do not routinely attempt to get the drug second checked? – this slice is completely removed.

The end result is that multiple defences have been weakened or removed and error is more likely, and the error is more likely to cause harm. Also be aware of the different types of error with potential gaps in knowledge, a latent/organisational error (no effective policy and possibly an issue with nurse staffing) and a routine violation.

14.5 Learning from error

Historically, those making mistakes have been identified and singled out for punishment and/or retraining, in what is often referred to as a culture of blame. With our example drug error blame would most likely have fallen on the shoulders of the individual administering and/or the doctor incorrectly prescribing. Does retraining these individuals make it safer for other or future patients? That clearly depends on the underlying reasons. If it was purely a knowledge gap, possibly, but does the same knowledge gap exist elsewhere? Potentially all the other issues remain unresolved. Moreover such punitive reactions make it less likely for individuals to admit mistakes and near misses in the future.

The focus is now on learning from error and, in shifting away from the individual, is much more focused on determining the system/organisational errors. Once robust systems, procedures and policies that work and are effective are in place, then errors can be captured. Of course issues will still need to be addressed where individuals have been reckless or lacked knowledge – but now reasons why the individuals felt the need to violate, or had not been given all the knowledge required, can be looked at.

For this to work health services need to learn from errors, adverse events and near misses. This requires engagement at both the individual level, by reporting errors, and the organisational level, investigating and feeding back the error using a systematic approach. It is also key that information is cascaded through the organisation and across the health service to raise awareness and prevent similar situations.

Violation may be indicative of the failure of systems, procedures or policies or other cultural issues. It is important that policies, procedures, roles and even our buildings and equipment are all designed pro-actively with human factors in mind so things do not have to be fixed retrospectively when adverse events occur. This means that all members of the organisation must be aware of human factors, not just the front-line clinical staff.

Improving team and individual performance

Having discussed the magnitude of the problem of healthcare error, the rest of this chapter will focus on how the performance of teams and individuals can be developed.

Raising awareness of the human factors and being able to practise these skills and behaviours within multi-professional teams allows the development of effective teams in all situations. Simulation activity allows a team to explore these new ideas, practise them and develop them. To do this we need feedback on our performance within a safe environment where no patient is at risk and egos and personal interests can be set aside. Consider how you developed a clinical skill. It was something that needed to be practised again and again until eventually it started to become automatic and routine. The same applies for our human factor behaviours. In addition, recognising our inherent human limitations and the situations when errors are more likely to occur, we can all be hyper-vigilant when required.

14.6 Communication

Poor communication is the leading cause of adverse events. This is not surprising; to have an effective team there needs to be good communication. The leader needs to communicate with the followers, and followers communicate with leaders and other followers. Communication is not just saying something – it is ensuring that information is accurately passed on and received. We all want to ensure effective communication at all times. Remember there are multiple components to effective communication (Table 14.2).

Table 14.2 Elements of communication				
Sender	**Sender**	**Transmitted**	**Receiver**	**Receiver**
Thinks of what to say	Says message	Through air, over phone, via email	Hears it	Thinks about it and acts

When communicating face-to-face a lot of the information is transmitted non-verbally, which can make telephone or email conversations more challenging. Communication can be more difficult when talking across professional, specialty or hierarchal barriers as we do not always talk the same technical language, have the same levels of understanding, or even have a full awareness of the other person's role.

There are a variety of similar tools to aid communication, like ATMIST and SBAR (Situation Background Assessment and Recommendation). Find out what your organisation uses and practise using it; look out for other staff using it too. These tools are designed for acute clinical communications. They facilitate the sender to plan and organise the message, make it succinct and focused, and provide it in a logical and expected order. They are also empowerment tools allowing the sender (who may be more junior) to request an action from a more senior individual. While these tools are useful, they tend to be reserved for certain situations, whereas we want to establish effective communication as the routine not the exception. One method to routinely improve communication is to incorporate a feedback loop.

Effective communication with a feedback loop

Errors can occur at any level or multiple levels. Consider a busy clinical situation and the team leader shouts *'We need an ECG connecting'* while looking at the blood pressure – what happens? The majority of times nothing – nobody goes to connect the ECG. So how can this be improved? Most obviously, an individual can be identified to perform the task, by name: *'Michael can you please connect the ECG?'* If Michael says *'yes'* effective communication might be assumed; but not always. What has Michael heard and what will he do? At the moment we do not really know what message has been received. Michael might dash over with a cup of tea as this is what he thought he heard. This may seem a slightly strange thing to happen; but how often in a clinical emergency have you asked for something and been presented with something else? People are less likely to ask questions in emergencies as everyone is busy. This could be the catalyst for an error or precipitate a missed task. So how do we find out what message Michael received? The easiest way is to include a feedback loop.

> Now the conversation goes:
>
> Team leader   'Michael, can you please connect the ECG?'
> Michael   'Okay, just connecting the ECG'

We now know that the message has been transmitted and received correctly. For this process to work both parties (the sender and receiver) need to understand and expect it – again demonstrating the need for us to practise and train together.

14.7 Team working, leadership and followership

At a basic level a team is a group of individuals with a common cause. Historically we have tended to train individually or in professional silos; the risk here is that we are making a 'team of experts' rather than an 'expert team'. Often within healthcare our teams form at short notice and often arrive at different times. Much emphasis has previously been given to the role of the leader, but a leader cannot be a team on his or her own. As much emphasis should be given to developing the other team members, the active followers. A good leader will be able to swap from the role of leader to follower as more senior staff arrive and agree to take over.

The leader

The leader's role is multifaceted and includes directing the team, assigning tasks and assessing performance, motivating and encouraging the team to work together, and planning and organising. All leadership skills and behaviours need to be developed and practised. There are different leadership styles and the leader needs to choose an appropriate style for that situation. Effective communication is key and should be reviewed and reflected upon regularly. Constructive feedback should both be given and sought in order to facilitate continuously improving performance.

Who is the leader?

It is vitally important to have a clearly identified leader. There can be times when people come and go, or different specialties arrive, creating a situation where it may not be clear who the leader is. In most organisations individuals will wear some form of identification to mitigate against this uncertainty. Documentation should record who is leading and any changes to the leader.

Physical position of the leader

As soon as the leader becomes hands on, and task focused, they are primarily concentrating on the task at hand. This becomes the focus of their thoughts and they lose situation awareness, their objective overview of the situation (see Section 14.8). The leader should be standing in an optimal position where they can gather all the information and ideally view the patient, the team members and the monitoring and diagnostic equipment. This enables them to recognise when a member is struggling with a task or procedure and support them appropriately.

Clear roles

It is important to introduce each other, and clarify roles and actions in emergencies. Sometimes this can be facilitated at the beginning of a shift but at other times it is impossible to predict or arrange. It is important, therefore, that individuals identify themselves to the leader as they arrive and roles are agreed, allocated and understood. A lot of the time their role may be determined purely in relation to the specific bleep the individual carries, but it is important that team members are flexible, for example if three airway providers are first on the scene we would expect other tasks to also be undertaken.

Followership

The followers have roles that are as mission critical as the leader. Followers are expected to work within their scope of practice and take the initiative. It is important to think about the level of communication required between the leader and followers. If it is obvious we are doing a task, this does not need to be communicated. There is a risk that followers can overwhelm the leader with verbal communications where, in fact, the key is to communicate concerns or abnormal things. In the Formula

One pit lane during a tyre change, the crew communicate (visually) as tasks are completed; they also signal if they have a problem, they do not communicate every expected step.

Hierachy

Within the team there needs to be a hierarchy. This is the power gradient; the leader is at the top of this as the person coordinating, directing and making the decisions. However, this should not be absolute. There is much discussion in the literature about the degree of the hierarchical gradient. If it is too steep the leader has a massive position of power, his or her decisions are unquestionable and the followers blindly follow the orders. This is not safe because leaders are humans too and also make errors – their team is their safety net. Safe practice is achieved where the followers feel they can raise concerns or question instructions. This must always be understood by the leaders as much as by the followers. One way to reduce the hierarchy is for the leader to invite the team's thoughts and concerns, particularly around patient safety issues. It is also important for the follower to learn how to raise concerns appropriately.

One method that is sometimes used to raise concerns appropriately is PACE (probing, alerting, challenging or declaring an emergency). The probing question allows diplomacy and maintenance of the hierarchy whilst raising a point.

Stage	Level of concern
P – Probe	*I think you need to know what is happening*
A – Alert	*I think something bad might happen*
C – Challenge	*I know something bad will happen*
E – Emergency	*I will not let it happen*

These stages are described with examples below:

- **Probe** – this is used where a person notices something they think might be a problem. They verbalise the issue, often as a question. 'Have you noticed that this child is cyanosed?'
- **Alert** – the observer strengthens and directs their statement and suggests a course of action. 'Dr Brown, I am concerned, the child is deeply cyanosed, should we start BVM ventilation?'
- **Challenge** – the situation requires urgent attention. One of the key protagonists needs to be directly engaged. If possible the speaker places him- or herself into the eye line of the person they wish to communicate with. 'Dr Brown, you must listen to me now, this patient needs help with his ventilation.'
- **Emergency** – this is used where all else has failed and/or the observer perceives a critical event is about to occur. Where possible a physical signal or physical barrier should be employed together with clear verbalisation. 'Dr Brown, you are overlooking this child's respiratory state, please move out of the way as I am going to ventilate him.'

The PACE structure can be commenced at any appropriate level and escalated until a satisfactory response is gained. If an adverse event is imminent then it may be relevant to start at the declaring 'emergency' stage, whereas a much lower level of concern may well start at a 'probing' question.

Some industries have also additionally adopted organisation-wide critical phrases that convey the importance of the situation, e.g. 'I am concerned', 'I am uncomfortable' or 'I am scared'.

14.8 Situation awareness

A key element of good team working and leadership is to be fully aware of what is happening; this is termed situation awareness. It not only involves seeing what is happening, but also captures how this is interpreted and understood, how decisions are made and ultimately to plan ahead.

Typically, three levels of situation awareness are described:

Level 1 – What is going on?
Level 2 – So what?
Level 3 – Now what?

Consider **Level 1** – the basic level – we are prone to errors even at this level. This is an active process, the risk seen is what is expected to be seen, rather than what is there. Figure 14.2 shows the similar package design of two different medications, making errors more likely. It is important to really concentrate on seeing what is actually there.

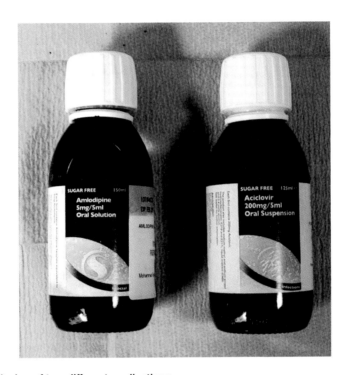

Figure 14.2 Similar package design of two different medications

Distraction

Within healthcare, distractions become the norm to such an extent individuals are often not even aware of them. The risk is that mistakes are made and information is missed. It is important to try to challenge interruptions when doing critical tasks, and when they do occur restart the task from the beginning, rather than from where it is considered the interruption occurred. Some organisations are looking at specific quiet areas for critical tasks. Whatever the local set up, the key is to develop and maintain everyone's awareness of how distraction greatly increases the chance of error.

Level 2 captures how someone's understanding forms from what has been seen. To minimise level 2 errors consideration is needed as to how the human brain works, recognises things and makes decisions and choices. This level of detail is beyond the scope of this chapter, and therefore this section will focus on a part of this – the decision making that leads into Level 3.

On the face of it the practice of decision making is familiar to everyone. However, to understand the factors that can compromise this process it is important to understand the factors that will influence the decision made. To make a good decision a person needs to assess all aspects of a problem, identify the possible responses to the problem, consider the consequences of each of those responses and then weigh up the advantages and disadvantages in order to draw a conclusion. Having completed this, they then need to communicate their decision to their team.

Good situation awareness is a basic prerequisite of this process. To achieve this, the decision maker must ensure they have all the key information. The whole team should be on the alert for ambiguities or conflicting information. Any inconsistent facts should be treated as a potential marker for faulty situation awareness. They should never be brushed off as unimportant anomalies in the absence of evidence to support such a decision.

In many clinical situations there can be a significant pressure of time. Where this is not the case then no decision-making process should be concluded until the team is satisfied they have all the information and have considered all the options. Where time is a pressure, a certain amount of pragmatism must be employed. There is plenty of evidence to confirm that practise and experience can mitigate some of the negative effects of abbreviating a decision-making process. Those making decisions under such circumstances need to remain aware of the short-cuts they have taken. They should be ready to receive feedback from their team, particularly if any member of the team has significant concerns about the proposed course of action.

Level 3 – having seen and understood we can now plan forward and communicate this with the team.

Team situation awareness

The individuals in the team may have a differing awareness of the situation depending on their previous experience, specialty, physical position, etc. The team's situation awareness will often be greater than any one individual's, however this can only be exploited if the individual elements are effectively communicated. The leader should actively encourage this.

14.9 Improving team and individual performance

In addition to effective communication, team working, situation awareness, leadership and followership skills, there are a number of other ways that team and individual performance can be further developed and improved.

Awareness of situations when errors are more likely

If we are aware that an error is more likely we can be more proactive in detecting them. Two common situations that make errors more likely are stress and fatigue. Stress is not only a source of error when we are overworked and overstimulated, but also, at the other end of the spectrum, when we are understimulated we become inattentive.

The acronym HALT has been used to describe situations when error is more likely:

H – Hungry
A – Angry
L – Late
T – Tired

IMSAFE has been used as a checklist in the aviation industry, asking whether the individual may be affected by:

I – Illness
M – Medication
S – Stress
A – Alcohol
F – Fatigue
E – Emotion

Ideally, individuals who are potentially compromised need to be supported appropriately, allowed time to recover and the team made aware. How this can be achieved in the middle of a night shift can be problematic.

Awareness of error traps

A common trap that people fall into is only seeing or registering the information that fits in with their current mental model. This is known as a *confirmation bias*. When this occurs people favour information that confirms their preconceptions or hypotheses regardless of whether the information is true. This may be observed within the healthcare setting during the process of a referral or handover. An example of this might be a clinician receiving clinical information as part of the call out. The clinician is advised that the patient is a known asthmatic. On their way to the patient's location, the clinician builds up a series of preconceived expectations around what they will find upon their arrival. They may even formulate a management plan whilst travelling to the scene, based upon their expectations. Once this mindset is established it can be difficult to shift.

On arrival, the clinician examines the systems affected by the presumed diagnosis. They seek to confirm their expectation by focusing on an auscultation of the chest at the expense of a thorough assessment. Upon hearing bilateral wheeze their preconceived ideas are confirmed and the remainder of the assessment is completed without due attention and more as a rehearsed exercise rather than an open-minded exploration. They fail to notice that the patient also has a soft stridor and is hypotensive. In this case the eventual diagnosis of anaphylaxis becomes at best a very late consideration, or at worst a situation that requires an objective newcomer to the team to point out the obvious.

Cognitive aids: checklists, guidelines and protocols

Cognitive aids such as guidelines are important because the human memory is not infallible. They also confer team understanding through the use of a standardised response. This reduces stress. This is especially true where an uncommon emergency event occurs. The team may be unfamiliar with one another and each member will be trying to remember what to do, what treatments are required and in what order. A good team leader will use the available cognitive aids as a prompt and the team's members can use it as a resource so that they can plan ahead. Safe practice is promoted through the use of these tools in an emergency rather than relying on memory.

Calling for help early

Trainee staff are often reluctant to call for senior help, partly due to not recognising the severity of the situation and partly due to concerns about wasting the time of seniors. With all emergency events, and in particular with paediatric emergencies, escalation and appropriate help should be summoned as soon as possible. Remember, help will not arrive instantly.

Using all available resources

Team resources include staff, observations, equipment, cognitive aids and the facilities in the local area. The team leader should continually consider the appropriateness of utilising available, un-tasked staff or equipment to optimise the patient's care and prevent a bottleneck in the treatment pathway.

Debriefing

Wherever possible a debriefing should be facilitated, even briefly, following clinical events. Ideally this should be normal procedure, rather than being reserved for catastrophic events. The aim of a debrief is to summarise any particular issues or problems that the team had, and reflect on how the team performed. Some organisations have set templates to facilitate this. It gives the opportunity for individuals, teams and organisations to continually develop.

14.10 Summary

In this chapter we have given a brief introduction to the human factors that can lead to poor team working, patient harm and adverse events. It is really important for you to use every opportunity to reflect and develop your own performance and influence the development of others and the team. Appropriate debriefing is included in the scenarios for the PHPLS course, which may be used to inform incorporation of this process into your own clinical practice.

CHAPTER 15
Practical procedures: airway and breathing

Learning outcomes

After reading this chapter, you will be able to identify the equipment for and describe the following procedures:
- Provision of supplementary oxygen
- Airway suction
- Oropharyngeal and nasopharyngeal airway insertion
- Mouth to mask ventilation
- Bag and mask ventilation
- Supraglottic airway device insertion
- Blocked tracheostomy management

15.1 Introduction

Following the control of catastrophic haemorrhage, the management of airway and breathing has the next priority in the resuscitation of patients of all ages. This chapter will discuss some of the skills required to manage the paediatric airway and provide oxygenation and ventilation. It will refer to but not discuss pre-hospital anaesthesia and endotracheal intubation.

> It should be stressed that basic airway manoeuvres are effective, and therefore life saving. Prolonged or repeated attempts at advanced airway techniques that interrupt ventilation and oxygenation or other on-going resuscitation will be detrimental.

15.2 Airway and breathing management: basic principles

Primary assessment and resuscitation

As discussed in Chapter 4, this consists of a rapid examination to identify immediately life-threatening emergencies. It is summarised as follows:

- Maintain an open airway
- Look, listen and feel
- Assess the effort of breathing
- Assess the efficacy of breathing
- Assess the effects of breathing

Pre-Hospital Paediatric Life Support: A Practical Approach to Emergencies, Third Edition. Edited by Alan Charters, Hal Maxwell and Paul Reavley.
© 2017 John Wiley & Sons Ltd. Published 2017 by John Wiley & Sons Ltd.

If a life-threatening airway or ventilation problem is identified, management of that problem should be performed immediately. After appropriate interventions have been performed, and their effect assessed, primary assessment is resumed or repeated.

Initial management

Airway

- Perform basic airway opening manoeuvres
- Provide suction if necessary
- Place airway adjuncts if necessary
- Proceed to advanced airway management if required and trained
- Should a cervical collar have been placed it should be loosened or removed if it impairs airway management (see Chapter 6 for guidance on cervical spine immobilisation)

Breathing

- Give high-flow oxygen
- Establish adequate ventilation if necessary with a bag–valve–mask and supplemental oxygen
- Decompress the stomach with a large-bore orogastric or nasogastric tube if necessary
- Perform chest decompression if necessary
- Monitoring: oxygen saturation monitoring (pulse oximetry), along with capnometry in a ventilated patient

Secondary assessment

This consists of a more thorough physical examination, together with appropriate investigations. Before embarking on this phase, it is important that the initial resuscitative measures are fully under way.

From the respiratory viewpoint, do the following, without causing undue delay:

- A more detailed examination of the airway, neck and chest
- Identify any swelling, bruising or wounds
- Re-examine for symmetry of chest movement and air entry
- Do not forget the back of the chest

Emergency treatment

If at any time the patient deteriorates, return to the primary assessment and re-cycle through the system, with any emergency interventions as required.

Team aspects of airway management

Resuscitation will be performed as part of a team of two or more. The 'team' will include professionals, but may also include a parent or other carer who may be able to help. Airway and breathing management will be undertaken by the most skilled in that role. As this involves taking a position at the head of the patient, the person in charge of the airway will also be in charge of protecting and managing the cervical spine if this is thought to be necessary. They will have a key role in the coordination of any rolling manoeuvres during the secondary survey, and in any subsequent transfer of the patient to an extrication device. Being at the patient's head, they will be in a position to see any significant untreated scalp lacerations, which can be a cause of significant blood loss in children.

Should the team be appropriately trained, the decision to start advanced airway techniques will be taken in full discussion with other team members. Depending on the number in the team, preparation for this may take place while other members of the team complete their part of the secondary survey. However, the actual performance of an advanced airway intervention is likely to involve at least one other person assisting.

Some severely injured or unwell children may benefit from pre-hospital anaesthesia and endotracheal intubation in order to commence early critical care. This is the preserve of specially trained teams and must not be undertaken without the correct training and competencies. Many countries have pre-hospital critical care teams who can either primarily respond or attend at the first responder's request. If this resource is not available then pre-hospital practitioners must persist with their own skill set and resources and transfer immediately.

Sequence of airway and breathing management

Assess the airway and give oxygen (A)

If dealing with a trauma case:

- Control of major haemorrhage occurs simultaneously
- Also consider cervical spine injury but do not allow this to significantly delay or interfere with essential airway management

If evidence of obstruction or altered consciousness:

- Perform airway opening manoeuvre (chin lift or jaw thrust if cervical spine injury is suspected)
- Suction secretions or blood under direct vision
- Foreign body removal if accessible
- Ventilate if no spontaneous or inadequate breathing and call for skilled support

If obstruction persists:

- Insert an airway adjunct – oropharygeal or nasopharyngeal
- Call for skilled support

If the airway is still obstructed:

- Reposition
- Try a two-person technique
- Try a supraglottic airway device

If obstruction still persists:

- Start advanced airway management if trained

Assess the breathing (B)

If breathing is inadequate:

- Ventilate with oxygen by bag and mask
- Consider supraglottic airway device if trained
- Continuous pulse oximetry and capnometry if ventilated
- Monitor for gastric insufflation and consider decompression with a nasogastric tube

Proceed to the rest of your primary survey

If patient deteriorates reassess airway and breathing

15.3 Equipment for providing oxygen and ventilation

Oxygen source

In the pre-hospital setting, oxygen supply is likely to be from cylinders. During daily checks it is important to make sure that you have sufficient oxygen.

Oxygen masks

Masks for spontaneous breathing

If available a mask with a reservoir bag should be used in the first instance so that a high concentration of oxygen can be delivered. A simple mask may be used later if a high oxygen concentration is no longer required (Figure 15.1). Small, frightened children may not well tolerate oxygen masks, in which case a parent may be able to help in holding the mask close, but not directly on, the face, or by simply wafting oxygen from the end of the oxygen tubing.

Some patients with chronic conditions may have home oxygen via nasal prongs. These are generally well tolerated, but they may cause drying of the airway, hence flow rates are limited. If these patients deteriorate they may require higher concentrations of oxygen, so the prongs should be replaced with a face mask.

Nebulisers may be fitted into the oxygen supply to enable inhaled drugs to be delivered, such as salbutamol, steroid and adrenaline (Figure 15.2). This should be driven at 8 l/min.

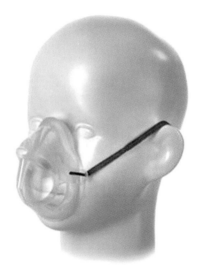

Figure 15.1 Simple face mask

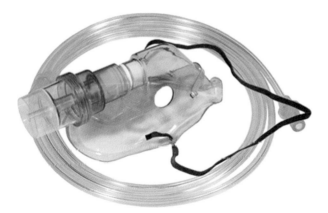

Figure 15.2 Oxygen mask with nebuliser

Face masks for artificial ventilation

Face masks for mouth-to-mouth or bag–valve–mask ventilation in infants are of two main designs (Figure 15.3). Some masks are shaped to conform to the anatomy of the child's face and have a low dead space. Circular, soft plastic masks give a good seal and are easier to use and preferred by many. Clear masks allow the presence of vomit to be seen, and also misting during effective ventilation.

The pocket mask is a single-size, clear plastic mask with a cushioned rim designed for mouth-to-mask resuscitation. It is usually supplied flattened in a rigid case, and needs pushing out into shape before use. It may have a port for attaching to an oxygen supply and can be used in adults and children. By using it upside down it may be used to ventilate an infant, flattening the more pointed end under the patient's chin.

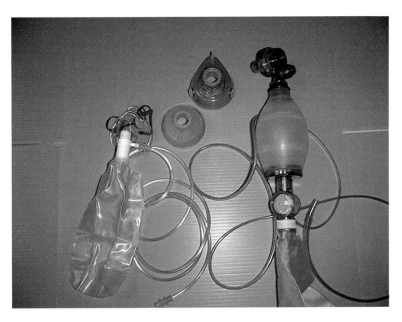

Figure 15.3 Face masks, bag–valve–mask and oxygen mask with reservoir

15.4 Basic airway management

Suction

Suction may be required to remove saliva, blood or vomit. Blind suctioning of the airway with a rigid suction device may cause injury to the oropharynx. Suction should be performed under direct vision. Prolonged suction in infants where the pharynx is excessively stimulated may also cause bradycardia.

A variety of suction devices are available. Most pre-hospital services will rely on portable battery-powered suction units that can be kept on charge in the vehicle. These can be backed up with hand-operated suction devices in case of failure (Figure 15.4); however the size of the suction tubing with these devices is often too large for infants.

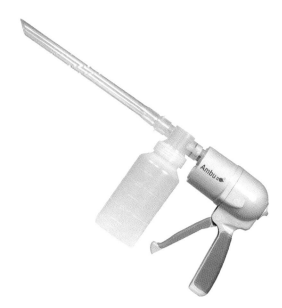

Figure 15.4 Example of a hand-powered suction unit with some control of suction pressure, and with interchangeable suction catheters (adult and paediatric)

Airway management with adjuncts

Basic techniques (chin lift or jaw thrust) are the core techniques and are usually successful in improving the airway in cases of obtunded consciousness. Only in some cases are adjuncts necessary.

Any equipment should be available in a variety of sizes, from infant to adult. Complete familiarity with airway equipment should be gained before an emergency occurs, and it should be checked before use.

Assessment and continued monitoring is a vital part of the safe use of an airway device, and appropriate equipment for this should also be available.

Pharyngeal airways

There are two main types of pharyngeal airway:

- Oropharyngeal
- Nasopharyngeal

Oropharyngeal airway

An oropharyngeal airway, otherwise referred to simply as an oral airway, or Guedel airway after its developer, may be used in the unconscious or obtunded patient for short-term airway management. It is frequently used as the first intervention when a patent airway cannot be achieved by the basic manual methods.

It provides a patent airway channel between the tongue and the posterior pharyngeal wall. It may also be used to stabilise the position of an oral endotracheal tube following intubation. It is only to be used in unconscious patients. In a patient with an intact gag reflex it will not be tolerated; do not attempt forced insertion as it may cause vomiting. During use if the patient begins to gag as the level of consciousness improves, the airway should be removed, or the patient allowed to remove it.

A correctly sized airway when placed vertically with its flange at the level of the incisors, will reach the angle of the mandible (Figure 15.5). This method of sizing is an estimate only, and a larger or smaller airway should be tried if no immediate improvement is seen. Too small an airway may be ineffective, too large an airway may cause laryngospasm. Either may cause oral trauma or may worsen airway obstruction.

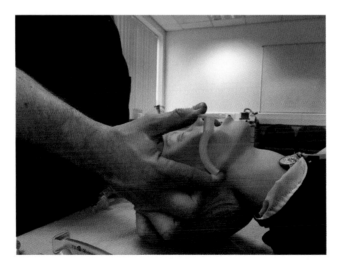

Figure 15.5 Sizing an oropharyngeal airway

Oropharyngeal airway (Guedel) insertion

1. Select the appropriate size by measuring vertically from the first incisor to the angle of the jaw.
2. Extend the neck slightly if safe to do so and open the mouth. In trauma patients open the mouth with a jaw thrust, avoiding excessive neck movement. (However, remember that in most resuscitations hypoxia is of greater risk to the patient than slight neck movement.)

3. Experienced practitioners can insert the airway upside down and then, when the airway is approximately half-way in, it is quickly rotated through 180° as it is passed over the tongue and soft palate taking care not to injure the soft tissues.
4. For inexperienced practitioners it is safer to insert the right way up, particularly for infants. The use of a tongue depressor or laryngoscope blade may aid insertion, so the airway just slides into place all the way in the correct orientation. When in position, the curve of the Guedel follows the natural curve of the tongue and pharynx (Figure 15.6), and the airway will sit naturally in place, with the flange just above the lip.
5. Be prepared to change to a different size if no airway improvement is achieved.
6. Remove the airway if the patient's level of consciousness improves and/or any gagging/choking occurs.

(a)   (b)   (c)

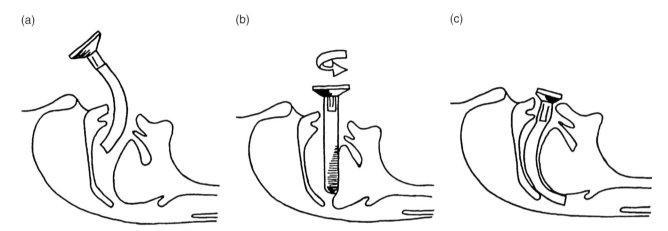

Figure 15.6 Airway insertion using the rotational technique

Nasopharyngeal airway

A nasopharyngeal airway is often better tolerated than a Guedel airway and may be left in place as the patient's level of consciousness improves. Insertion may cause nose bleeds, especially if it is not well lubricated. It may be possible to insert a nasopharyngeal airway when it is not possible to open the mouth sufficiently to insert an oral airway (e.g. a fitting child with tight clenching of the jaw).

It is contraindicated in fractures of the anterior base of the skull. (Look for signs such as peri-orbital bruising, or Battle's sign (bruising over the mastoid).) However, as always, the airway takes priority.

A suitable length can be estimated by measuring from the lateral edge of the nostril to the tragus of the ear (Figure 15.7). An appropriate diameter is one that just fits into the nostril without causing blanching (Figure 15.8). Remember that these sizing guidelines are just estimates, be prepared to change to a differently sized tube if necessary.

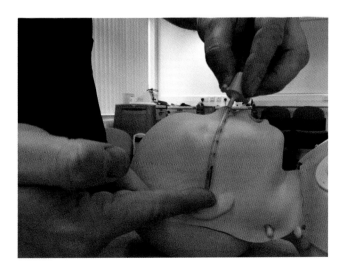

Figure 15.7 Sizing a nasopharyngeal airway: length

If small-sized nasopharyngeal airways are not available, shortened endotracheal tubes may be used. Use a large safety pin to prevent loss into the nose.

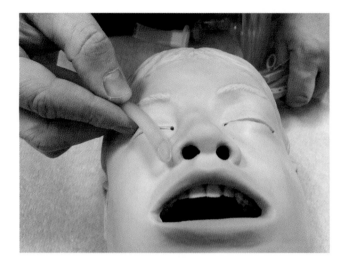

Figure 15.8 Sizing a nasopharyngeal airway: diameter

Nasopharyngeal airway insertion

1. Select the appropriate size.
2. Lubricate the airway with a water-soluble lubricant.
3. Insert the tip into the nostril and direct it posteriorly along the floor of the nose towards the tragus and not the forehead (Figure 15.9).
4. Gently pass the airway past the turbinates with a to-and-fro rotating motion. As the tip advances into the pharynx, a palpable 'give' may be felt.
5. Continue until the flange rests on the nostril.
6. If there is difficulty inserting the airway, consider using the other nostril or a smaller size from the original estimate. Do not use excessive force or have repeat attempts.
7. Reassess airway and breathing, provide oxygen and commence ventilation if necessary.

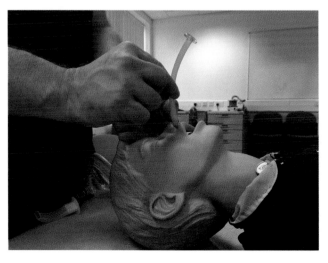

Figure 15.9 Nasopharyngeal insertion

Mouth-to-mask ventilation

1. Pocket masks and similar devices will need pushing into shape before use.
2. A filter, if present, may be attached to the mask before use.
3. It is usual to use both hands to hold the mask. Apply the mask to the face, using a jaw thrust grip, the thumbs holding the mask. If using a shaped mask, it should be the right way up in children (Figure 15.10) or upside down in infants (Figure 15.11). Ensure a neutral head position in infants, more extended in older children.
4. Ensure an adequate seal.
5. Blow into the mouth port, observing the resulting chest movement. Do not give excessive tidal volumes.
6. Ventilate at an initial 12–20 breaths per minute, depending on the age of the child. If using the mask for cardiopulmonary resuscitation (CPR) then use two ventilations to 15 compressions.
7. Attach oxygen to the face mask if possible.

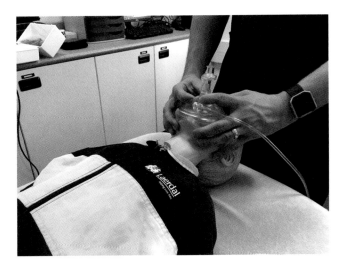

Figure 15.10 Mask position for mouth-to-mask ventilation in a child

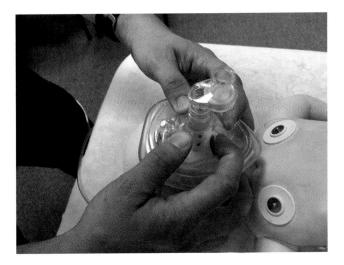

Figure 15.11 Mask position for mouth-to-mask ventilation in an infant

Gastric tubes

Children are prone to air swallowing and vomiting. Air may also be forced into the stomach during bag and mask ventilation. This may cause regurgitation, vagal stimulation and diaphragmatic splinting, which can prevent adequate ventilation. A gastric tube will decompress the stomach and significantly improve both breathing and general well-being. Withholding the procedure 'to be kind to the child' may cause more distress than performing it. Good fixation is needed to prevent displacement.

Bag and mask ventilation

> Bag and mask ventilation with a self-inflating bag is absolutely the core skill of emergency airway and breathing management.

It may appear to be simple and routine. In fact it is a skill that takes practice and experience to acquire; this applies particularly to single operator use.

Self-inflating bags

Self-inflating bags come in three sizes: typically about 250, 500 and 1500 ml, depending on the manufacturer. The smallest bag is ineffective except in very small babies, so the choice is usually between the two larger sizes. Especially in the two smaller sizes, bags often have a pressure-limiting valve set at 4.5 kPa (45 cmH$_2$O). This valve protects normal lungs from inadvertent high-pressure ventilation trauma ('barotrauma'). The valve may occasionally need to be overridden for high resistance (low compliance) lungs. Beware, however – technique needs to be good in this situation, as forced ventilation via a face mask at high pressure is more likely to cause gastric inflation unless carefully performed.

The patient end of the self-inflating bag connects to the face mask via a one-way valve of a fish-mouth or leaf-flap design. The opposite end has a connection to the oxygen supply and to a reservoir attachment. The reservoir enables high oxygen concentrations to be delivered. Without a reservoir bag, it is difficult to supply more than 50% oxygen to the patient whatever the fresh gas flow; whereas with a reservoir bag and high-flow oxygen, an inspired oxygen concentration of over 95% can be achieved. Should the oxygen supply fail, ventilation can still continue, but with air.

Technique

1. Apply the mask to the face. The thumb and first finger are placed on top of the mask; the third and fourth fingers perform a chin lift, and the fifth finger a jaw thrust (Figure 15.12). The jaw and chin need to be pulled up to the mask to obtain a seal. Pushing the mask down into the face results in neck flexion and obstructs the airway.
2. Squeeze the bag, looking for chest movement, misting of the mask and end-tidal CO$_2$ if available. If the chest is not moving, consider:
   - adjusting the head extension to one appropriate to the size of the patient
   - repositioning the mask
   - using an airway adjunct
   - employing a two-person technique
3. Ventilate at approximately 20 breaths per minute or a ratio of two ventilations to 15 chest compression if performing CPR.
4. The bag should be connected to an oxygen supply at 15 l/min.
5. Continually reassess the efficacy of ventilation and oxygenation.
6. Do not overventilate. Overenthusiastic ventilation, with excessive tidal volumes or very rapid inspirations, may force gas into the stomach. The resulting gastric distension will inhibit ventilation, and also encourage regurgitation.

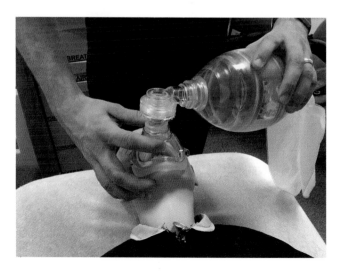

Figure 15.12 Bag and mask ventilation

A two-person technique (Figure 15.13) makes obtaining a seal around the mask easier, with both hands of one rescuer holding the mask. The thumbs are used on top of the mask and the first fingers used to perform a jaw thrust. Holding the mask is the job for a skilled person. The other rescuer, who may be less skilled, supports and squeezes the bag. In conjunction with an oropharyngeal airway, this is an extremely effective method for airway management in an unconscious, apnoeic patient.

However, it does occupy two persons (potentially all of a two-person crew if no other assistance is available), so single-handed bag–mask ventilation is the core skill that should be acquired and practised.

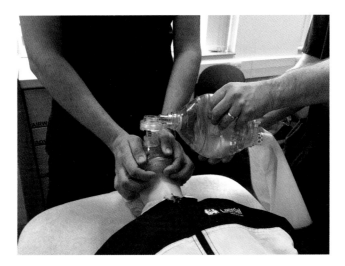

Figure 15.13 Two-person bag and mask ventilation

15.5 Advanced airway and breathing techniques

Breathing systems

For manual ventilation before or during transportation, via a face mask, supraglottic airway or endotracheal tube, the self-inflating bag is the commonest and most reliable technique, as it needs no power source other than the operator's hand, and can function with air should the oxygen supply fail.

Note on home ventilation

Some children may be on long-term home ventilation. Ventilation may be full time or nocturnal only. Ventilation may be through a close fitting face mask or a tracheostomy. Generally, home ventilators are very reliable. An example is shown in Figure 15.14.

Parents or other long-term carers will be more experienced in the use of these ventilators than many practitioners, whether pre-hospital or hospital based. If problems have arisen with home ventilation via a tracheostomy, follow the usual systematic approach. Airway first, then breathing (i.e. check tracheostomy for patency and position first, with suctioning, then use of self-inflating bag to replace the home ventilator).

Should high concentrations of oxygen be required, replace the home ventilator with a self-inflating bag with reservoir.

Supraglottic airway devices

Supraglottic airway devices (SADs) are commonly used in both hospital and pre hospital care. There two main devices used in the UK – the laryngeal mask airway (LMA), which has an inflatable cuff that forms a seal at the laryngeal inlet, and the i-gel, which has a firm gel-like cuff which does not require inflation and is stiffer when inserted.

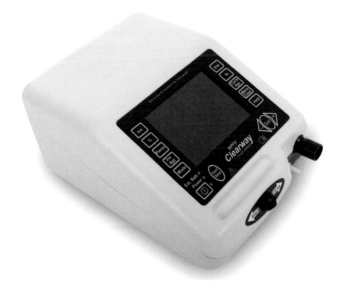

Figure 15.14 Home ventilator. Source: nippyventilator.com. Reproduced with permission of B&D Electromedical

The LMA has an inflatable elliptical mask that sits around the laryngeal inlet. At the proximal end is a tube similar to a large endotracheal tube, with a pilot tube to inflate the cuff. The original LMAs were reusable, but disposable LMAs and other designs such as the intubating LMA are now available, some designs incorporating a channel for suctioning of gastric contents.

LMAs have some advantages:

- Are quick and easy to insert, even if the operator is inexperienced
- Allow one-handed or hands-free ventilation (if attached to a ventilator)
- Provide some protection of the airway from aspiration. Note: they are not, however, considered a definitive airway
- Reduce the amount of gastric insufflation
- May have an inbuilt suction channel to enable gastric suction and decompression

Both LMAs and i-gels are available in paediatric sizes (Tables 15.1 and 15.2).

Training in the use of supraglottic airways is still advisable, as it is still possible for them to be mis-placed. Success rates are very high in those experienced in their use, although lower in infants.

Note that the manufacturers' recommended sizes for different patient weights differ slightly between LMAs and i-gels.

Table 15.1 Laryngeal mask airway (LMA) sizes		
Patient weight (kg)	LMA size (standard disposable LMA)	Max. cuff vol (ml)
<5	1	5
5–10	1.5	7
10–20	2	10
20–30	2.5	15
30–50	3	20
50–70	4	30
>70	5	40

Excepting the two smallest sizes, maximum cuff inflation volume is given by the formula:

Approx. inflation volume (ml) = (LMA size × 10) − 10

Note: recommended maximum inflation volumes vary slightly between different manufacturers and models of LMA. Check packaging.

Table 15.2 i-gel sizes

Patient weight (kg)	i-gel size
<5	1
5–12	1.5
10–25	2.0
25–35	2.5
30–60	3
50–90	4
90+	5

Insertion of the classic LMA

The insertion of LMAs is rapid, and blind (i.e. no laryngoscopy is required). LMAs can easily become displaced, however, and may rotate as the LMA tube is round. They do not protect completely from aspiration.

Equipment

- Appropriate size LMA
- Syringe for LMA cuff inflation
- Water-soluble lubricant
- Stethoscope
- Tape to secure LMA

Procedure

1. Administer oxygen and support ventilation whilst preparing to insert the LMA.
2. Check the LMA, in particular checking cuff inflation with no leak, and check the tube for blockage or loose objects; have lubricant and suction to hand.
3. Deflate the cuff and lightly lubricate the back and sides of the mask. Avoid excessive amounts of lubricant. In children, it may be preferred to have the cuff partially inflated for insertion.
4. Tilt the patient's head back (if safe to do so), open the mouth fully, and insert the tip of the mask along the hard palate with the open side facing, but not touching, the tongue (Figure 15.15a). A jaw thrust performed by an assistant, if available, may aid placement.
5. Slide the mask further, along the posterior pharyngeal wall, with your index finger initially providing support for the tube (Figure 15.15b). Eventually resistance is felt as the tip of the LMA lies at the upper end of the oesophagus (Figure 15.15c).
6. Fully inflate the cuff. The LMA should be seen to rise up slightly as it is inflated.
7. Ventilate and check its position as for a tracheal tube: good equilateral chest rise, no leak, capnometry if available. If not ventilating adequately, remove and return to bag–valve–mask ventilation whilst preparing a second attempt.
8. If adequately ventilating, secure the LMA with adhesive tape.

It is sometimes easier to insert an LMA rotated 90°, or 180°, from its final position. The mask is then quickly rotated into its natural position as it passes though the oropharynx. If the cuff is folding, rotating or catching, partial inflation prior to insertion may resolve this.

Complications of LMA use

- The epiglottis can get caught by the LMA and displaced over the larynx. This results in obstruction of the airway
- The tip of the LMA may fold over during insertion
- If either of the above problems occurs, or if the airway is unsatisfactory for another reason, withdraw the LMA and re-insert
- Rotation of LMAs may occur after insertion, more commonly with smaller LMAs and particularly while the breathing system or self-inflating bag is attached

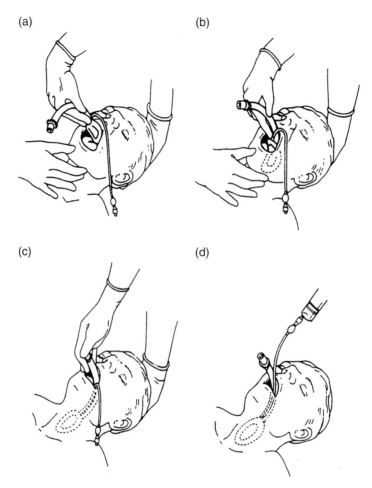

(a)　　　　　　　　(b)

(c)　　　　　　　　(d)

Figure 15.15 Insertion of the laryngeal mask airway

I-gel insertion

The principles of insertion are broadly similar to the LMA.

1. The i-gel is supplied in a protective cradle. A small blob of water-soluble lubricant jelly can be placed onto the cradle to facilitate light lubrication of the back, sides and front of the gel cuff.
2. The device is inserted into the mouth, sliding it backwards along the hard palate until a clear resistance is felt. It is not necessary to insert fingers into the patient's mouth during insertion.
3. A jaw thrust by the assistant may aid insertion if early resistance is felt, or, alternatively, insertion 'upside down' followed by rotation may aid insertion.

With both LMA and i-gel insertion, the device is in place when definitive resistance is felt.

Management of a blocked tracheostomy

See Figure 15.16.

Many children with an established tracheostomy will improve by removal of the blocked tube, allowing them to breathe through the stoma prior to replacing the blocked tube with a new one.

However, there are risks in removing the tube from a newly created tracheostomy as, until the stoma track is established, attempted replacement of a tracheostomy tube may be difficult and a blind-ending false track could be created. This is unlikely to be a problem in the pre-hospital setting, as patients with newly created tracheostomies will normally be kept in hospital until the stoma is well formed and stable.

Parents who routinely care for their child's tracheostomy at home may be more familiar with tube suction and tube changing for their child than pre-hospital personnel, or hospital staff in medical areas, where this is rarely performed.

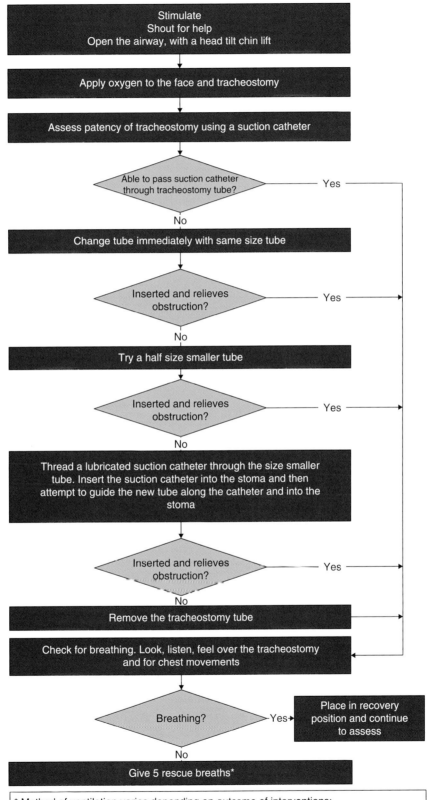

Figure 15.16 Management of a blocked tracheostomy

Procedure

Commence basic life support.

1. Stimulate the child.
2. Shout for help.
3. Open and check the airway, with a head tilt chin lift. This both exposes the tracheostomy tube and opens the upper airway.
4. Apply oxygen to the face and tracheostomy.
5. Assess patency of the tracheostomy using a suction catheter.
6. If you are unable to pass the suction catheter through the tracheostomy tube, then the tube must be changed immediately with the same size tube. If this fails to relieve the obstruction, or you cannot insert it:
   - try a half size smaller tube
   - if it is not possible to insert this, thread a lubricated suction catheter through the size smaller tracheostomy tube. Insert the suction catheter into the stoma and then attempt to guide the new tracheostomy tube along the catheter and into the stoma
   - if this is unsuccessful then remove the tracheostomy tube
7. Check for breathing. Look, listen, feel: place the side of your face over the tracheostomy tube and face to listen and feel for any breaths, and at the same time look at the child's chest to observe any breathing movement. If the child is breathing satisfactorily, place them in the recovery position and continue to assess. If the child is not breathing, you will have to give rescue breaths.
8. Give five rescue breaths.
9. If you have succeeded in removing the obstructed tracheostomy and replaced it with a patent tracheostomy tube you should attach a self-inflating bag and ventilate (or if that is not available, perform mouth-to-tracheostomy ventilation).
10. If you havfe failed to replace the tracheostomy tube:
    - if the child has a fully or partially patent upper airway, occlude the tracheal stoma and provide rescue breaths via the mouth by bag–valve–mask or mouth to mouth
    - if the child does not have a patent upper airway these resuscitation breaths are applied direct to the stoma

15.6 Summary

Following control of catastrophic haemorrhage, the management of airway and breathing has priority in the resuscitation of patients of all ages. The rate at which respiratory function can deteriorate in children is particularly high. Effective resuscitation techniques must be applied quickly and in order of priority.

CHAPTER 16
Practical procedures: circulation

Learning outcomes

After reading this chapter, you will be able to identify the equipment for and describe the following procedures:
- Peripheral venous access
- Intraosseus access
- Manual defibrillation

16.1 Vascular access

Access to the circulation is a crucial step in delivering care to a critically ill child. Many access routes are possible; the one chosen will reflect both clinical need and the skills of the operator.

If immediate drugs or fluids are required then vascular access should be secured at the scene. Patients travelling by air should have all necessary access prior to leaving as the rotary wing environment makes intravenous (IV) access very tricky. On road moves, it is possible to stop and gain access should it be suddenly needed. Securing the cannula and fluid and drug administration can be done in transit.

If timely venous access cannot be gained (within 2 minutes) or there have been two failed attempts, consider the intraosseous (IO) route.

Peripheral venous access

Try to avoid leaving a tourniquet on a child longer than is necessary. Tourniquets are uncomfortable and frightening. It is better, if possible, to ask a colleague to squeeze the limb with their hand rather than use a tourniquet. This will also assist in keeping the limb immobilised for needle insertion.

Veins on the dorsum of the hand, the antecubital fossa, are commonly used for access in children. In infants, veins in the foot are often used and the saphenous vein at the medial aspect of the ankle can be used for cannulation Standard percutaneous techniques should be employed, if possible. Always check the glucose level on any blood that flashes back on insertion.

Pre-Hospital Paediatric Life Support: A Practical Approach to Emergencies, Third Edition. Edited by Alan Charters, Hal Maxwell and Paul Reavley.
© 2017 John Wiley & Sons Ltd. Published 2017 by John Wiley & Sons Ltd.

Equipment

- Skin cleansing swabs
- Suitable sized cannula
- Extension set, flushed with 0.9% saline
- Syringe and 0.9% saline
- Adhesive tape

Procedure

1. Locate a vein.
2. Restrain the child.
3. Ask someone to squeeze the limb proximally or apply a tourniquet.
4. Clean the skin.
5. Insert the cannula and attach the three-way tap with flushed line.
6. Release the pressure on the limb (hand or tourniquet).
7. Secure the cannula with tape.
8. Flush the cannula via the three-way tap with 2–5 ml of saline and ensure there is no swelling around the site.
9. Commence drug administration or bolus fluid administration as required.

Intraosseous infusion

Because it is important to achieve vascular access quickly in many life-threatening situations, IO access is recommended when IV access attempts have failed. It is fast, easy and reliable. Modern assisted IO devices have made it a simple technique. It is indicated if other attempts at venous access fail, or if they will take longer than 2 minutes to carry out in a truly life-threatening clinical situation. However, for clinicians with no experience of paediatric cannulation IO access should be the first route in life-threatening conditions.

Unless the rescuer is experienced in paediatric intravenous cannulation, intraosseus should be the first choice for access in the severely ill or injured child.

Equipment

- Alcohol swabs
- Size 16 G IO needle with trochar (at least 1.5 cm in length)
- EZIO equipment drill and needle set
- 5 ml syringe
- Three-way tap with short extension set, flushed with 0.9% saline
- 20 ml syringe, or 50 ml syringe, as appropriate
- Infusion fluid

EZIO procedure

1. Identify the infusion site. Options include: below the tibial tuberosity; lateral femoral condyle; proximal humerus; and anterior iliac crest. The proximal humerus is especially useful to access if the lower limbs are unaccessible or proximal vascular injury is suspected. The various approaches to insertion will be covered in the skills station.
2. Clean the skin over the chosen site.
3. Insert the needle at 90° to the skin.
4. Drill the needle to the correct depth.
5. Aspirate for marrow, and check glucose.
6. Flush the needle firmly.
7. Attach the filled 50 ml syringe via a three-way tap and push in the infusion fluid in boluses.

Manual technique

1. Identify the infusion site. Fractured bones should be avoided, as should limbs with fractures proximal to possible sites. The landmarks for the upper tibial and lower femoral sites are shown in the box, and illustrated in Figure 16.1.
2. Clean the site. Use local anaesthesia if there is any degree of consciousness in the patient.
3. Insert the needle at 90° to the skin.
4. Continue to advance the needle using a twisting motion until a 'give' is felt as the cortex is penetrated.
5. Attach the 5 ml syringe and aspirate bone marrow to check position. If bone marrow cannot be aspirated, push in a few millilitres of normal saline; if this flows in easily, the needle is in the bone marrow.
6. Check glucose level on bone marrow aspirated.
7. Attach a three-way tap.
8. Push in fluid boluses as required. Gravity-dependent IV fluid administration sets will not flow via this route.
9. Immobilise the leg in an orange box splint (or similar) for easy identification.

Surface anatomy for intraosseous infusions

Tibial	*Femoral*
Anterior surface, 2–3 cm below and medial to the tibial tuberosity	Anterolateral surface, 3 cm above the lateral condyle

---

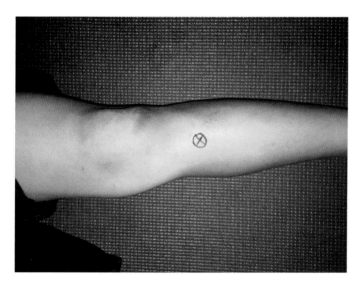

Figure 16.1 Tibial site for intraosseous infusion

16.2 Fluid management

Children with severe shock will require immediate fluids. Access should be gained at scene, if necessary intraosseous. If access is required during road transit, it is recommended that the vehicle is stopped whilst attempts are performed.

Fluid volume

The circulating volume in children is 80–90 ml/kg. Fluid boluses are calculated at 10 ml/kg with immediate reassessment, and administered as a fluid challenge to children with hypovolaemic shock due to medical conditions. Fluids should be given cautiously in trauma, diabetic ketoacidosis (DKA) and cardiac conditions. Overfilling can be dangerous and in these situations fluid should be given in 5 ml/kg boluses, repeated to effect.

Basic rules include the following:

-   Initial resuscitation should be with 0.9% NaCl or Hartmann's solution
-   All fluids should be warmed if possible
-   **Never use hypotonic/hyponatremic fluids for resuscitation**
-   Use a syringe and three-way tap to administer fluid – it is faster and more accurate. IO fluids MUST be given this way, gravity alone will not suffice.

- Draw up 10 ml/kg (5 ml/kg in trauma, cardiac diseases and DKA)
- Reassess after each bolus if 10% dextrose has been used to correct hypoglycaemia; do not count it as part of the volume used for resuscitation
- Keep accurate records of how much, what and when and provide good handover at the hospital

Diabetic ketoacidosis

A significant cause of death in DKA is cerebral oedema and it is believed that too rapid and/or too much IV fluid may be the reason. It is unusual to find a child who is shocked with DKA, even despite significant dehydration, because the fluid abnormalities have developed over a considerable time. It is therefore advised NOT to give any IV fluid to a child with DKA, unless they are exhibiting signs of significant shock. If this is the case, 5 ml/kg may be given. This may be repeated once if the shock remains significant. If the journey time is long (or retrieval is delayed) then further fluid should only be given on senior medical advice.

16.3 Manual defibrillation

In order to achieve the optimum outcome, defibrillation must be performed quickly and efficiently. This requires:

- Correct pad selection
- Correct pad placement
- Good pad contact
- Correct energy selection

Many defibrillators are available. The majority of new models use sticky pads to deliver the charge; older defibrillators may use paddles instead. Pre-hospital paediatric life support providers should make sure they are familiar with those they may have to use. Most automatic/semi-automatic defibrillators are not designed for use in children aged below 8 years (25 kg) because of the different energy requirements of children compared with adults. Manual defibrillators capable of appropriate energy adjustment and automated defibrillators specifically designed for children should therefore be used for younger children.

Correct pad selection

Most defibrillators are supplied with adult pads attached (13 cm diameter, or equivalent area); 4.5 cm diameter pads are suitable for use in infants, and 8 cm diameter should be used for small children (if available).

Correct pad placement

The usual placement is anterolateral. One pad is put over the apex in the mid-axillary line, and the other is placed just to the right of the sternum, immediately below the clavicle (Figure 16.2).

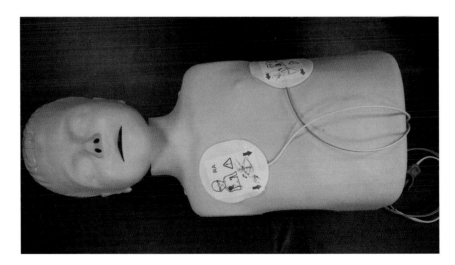

Figure 16.2 Anterolateral paddle placement

If the anteroposterior placement is used, one pad is placed just to the left side of the lower part of the sternum, and the other just below the tip of the left scapula (Figure 16.3). In an infant the pads will be placed as seen in Figure 16.3.

(a)   (b)

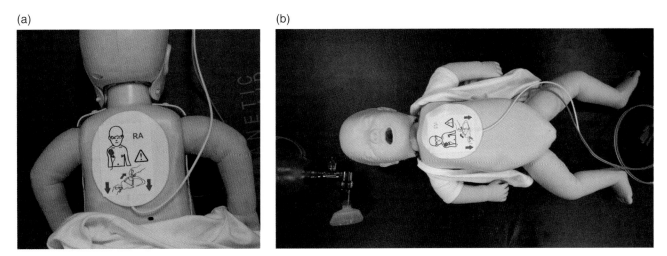

Figure 16.3 Anteroposterior pad placement in an infant

Good pad/paddle contact

Gel pads should always be used. Firm pressure should be applied to paddles if using.

Correct energy selection

The recommended levels are shown in Section 7.7.

Safety

A defibrillator delivers enough current to *cause* cardiac arrest. The user must ensure that other rescuers are not in either direct or indirect (pools of water, etc.) physical contact with the patient (or the trolley) at the moment the shock is delivered. The defibrillator should only be charged when the pads are correctly positioned on the child's chest.

> **Basic life support should be interrupted for the shortest possible time (see stages 4–9 below).**

Procedure (before commencing stop vehicle if necessary)

1. Confirm cardiac arrest.
2. Perform uninterrupted chest compressions.
3. Apply defibrillator adhesive pads.
4. Select the energy required (4 J/kg)
5. Ensure that the only person touching the child is the rescuer providing cardiac compressions.
6. Press the charge button.
7. Wait until the defibrillator is charged.
8. Tell all those around the patient to stand clear: shout, 'stand clear'.
9. Check that all other rescuers are clear.
10. Deliver the shock.
11. Recommence chest compressions for 2 minutes without checking rhythm.
12. Reassess the rhythm after 2 minutes, if ventricular fibrillation/pulseless ventricular tachycardia persist repeat stages 1–11 and deliver another shock.

CHAPTER 17
Practical procedures: trauma

Learning outcomes

After reading this chapter, you will be able to identify the equipment for and describe the following procedures:
- Sealing open chest wounds
- Needle decompression of the chest
- Finger thoroacostomy
- Spinal immobilisation
- Helmet removal

17.1 Sealing open chest wounds

An open pneumothorax can cause respiratory failure complicated by the entraining of air through the wound into the pleural space rather than through the trachea to the lungs. These wounds have been described as 'sucking chest wounds'. They are dealt with as part of the 'B' of the primary survey, after ensuring that catastrophic haemorrhage is controlled and the patient's airway is patent. The aim of treatment is to seal the wound with a dressing that allows air within the pleural space out during expiration, whilst preventing air being drawn back into the pleural space on inspiration. All penetrating chest wounds should be sealed with an appropriate dressing designed for this purpose. Dressing an open pneumothorax with an occlusive dressing can convert it to a tension pneumothorax.

Chest seals

Historically, open pneumothoraces (sucking chest wounds) have been closed using a square of plastic sealed on three sides, described as a three-sided dressing. However, with the availability of designed for-purpose commercial chest seals this method should only be used if there is no alternative. There are several types of chest seals commercially available, including the Asherman, Bolin and Russell chest seals (Figure 17.1). All work on the same premise by sealing the chest wound and employing a one-way valve principle to prevent a tension pneumothorax occurring.

Remember, whichever method you choose, it is vital you constantly reassess the patient's condition; if the patient's condition does deteriorate, this dressing should be checked and the child reassessed.

Pre-Hospital Paediatric Life Support: A Practical Approach to Emergencies, Third Edition. Edited by Alan Charters, Hal Maxwell and Paul Reavley.
© 2017 John Wiley & Sons Ltd. Published 2017 by John Wiley & Sons Ltd.

(a)   (b)

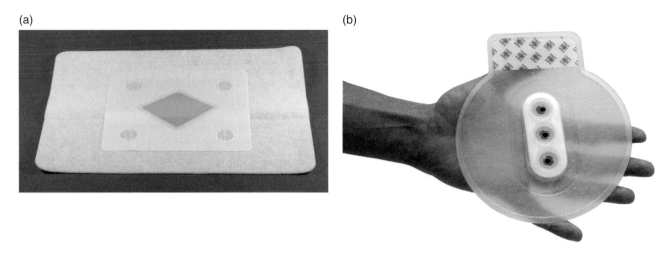

Figure 17.1 (a) Russell chest seal. Source Prometheus Medical. Reproduced with permission of Prometheus Medical. **(b) Bolin chest seal.** Source: H&H Medical Corp. Reproduced with permission of H&H Medical Corp.

17.2 Chest decompression

Needle thoracocentesis

This procedure to treat tension pneumothorax can be life saving and performed quickly with minimum equipment. Once performed, careful reassessment is required; if the patient 're-tensions', repeat the procedure. Ensure that the presence of the needle decompression is carefully handed over on arrival at hospital.

Minimum equipment

- Skin cleansing swabs
- Large over-the-needle intravenous cannula (largest available and possible)
- 5 or 10 ml syringe
- Adhesive tape

Procedure

1. Identify the second intercostal space in the mid-clavicular line (Figure 17.2) on the side of the pneumothorax (evidenced by diminished breath sounds; hyper-resonance on percussion compared to the unaffected side; and, in very late stages, tracheal deviation).
2. Swab the chest wall with surgical prep solution or a skin cleansing swab.
3. Attach the syringe to the rear port of the cannula.
4. Insert the cannula into the chest wall, just above the rib below, aspirating all the time (Figure 17.2).
5. Remove the needle, leaving the plastic cannula in place.
6. Secure the cannula in place and monitor the patient for signs of deterioration, repeat decompression if the childs' condition deteriorates. A secondary decompression site is the fourth or fifth intercostal space on the mid-axilliary line (see Figure 17.3).
7. If the patient is ventilated, the patient will require a finger thoracostomy and if the pre-hospital phase is prolonged, chest drain insertion.

> Needle thoracocentesis must be followed by chest drain placement in hospital.

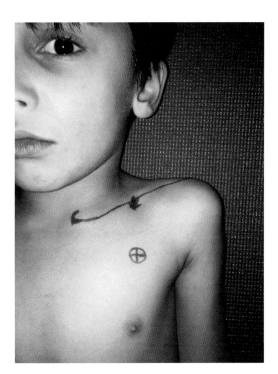

Figure 17.2 Needle thoracocentesis site

Finger thoracostomy

Ventilated patients with a suspected tension pneumothorax should be decompressed using a finger thoracostomy. Practitioners must be trained in this procedure.

Minimum equipment

- Skin cleansing swabs
- Disposable scalpel
- Blunt forceps

Procedure

1. On the affected side, abduct the arm to >90°, exposing the 'triangle of safety'. The triangle of safety is identified by the lateral border of the pectoralis major and the anterior border of the latissimus dorsi which meet at an apex in the axilla (Figure 17.3).
2. Swab the chest wall with surgical prep solution or a skin cleansing swab.
3. Identify the fourth or fifth intercostal space, anterior to the mid-axillary line, ensuring this falls within the triangle of safety.
4. Using a disposable scalpel, create a 3–4 cm incision into the subcutaneous tissue; the incision should follow the directions of the ribs.
5. Using a set of blunt forceps, dissect through the intercostal muscles and pleura, creating an aperture large enough to insert a finger through.
6. Whilst the forceps are still in position, insert your finger into the pleural space, ensuring an opening has been created. Withdraw the forceps.
7. Rotate your finger and sweep your finger clockwise and anticlockwise to feel for the lung or abdominal organs in the thoracic cavity, allowing air to escape.
8. Cover using a chest seal as described earlier.
9. Safely dispose of all equipment used in the procedure.

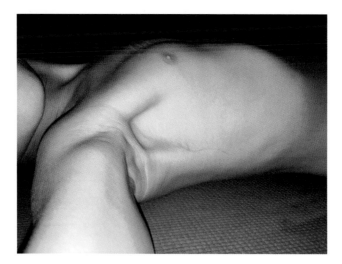

Figure 17.3 Triangle of safety

17.3 Spinal care

In a situation where there is a high index of suspicion of spinal injury, a child should initially be manually stabilised whilst immobilisation equipment is being prepared.

The long spinal board is an extraction device only; patients should never be transported on rigid boards. There are other transport devices available such as the scoop stretcher and vacuum mattresses.

The principle of minimal handling is advocated in keeping with clot preservation. The use of the correct immobilisation device pre-hospital supports this principle, and if correctly applied avoids unnecessary patient moving and handling later during the patient's care.

This minimal handling approach is not new, but builds on the evidence that the use of multiple equipment, frequent log rolling and change of equipment once at hospital can be detrimental to the patient.

Cervical spine immobilisation

Although the vast majority of paediatric trauma patients will probably not sustain significant cervical trauma, it is advisable to consider the presence of a spinal injury in all significantly injured children. It is only when adequate assessment and investigation has been carried out that the decision to remove cervical spine protection can be taken. This is not always possible to perform on the scene. It is well documented, however, that a conscious child with a significant cervical injury will be very aware of this, often reporting their fears before any assessment is started. Remember, cervical spine immobilisation should only be performed on cooperative patients and is not indicated in penetrating neck injuries.

Hard cervical collars are no longer advocated in children. If spinal immobilisation is required, the first step is manual in-line stabilisation (Figure 17.4). This is maintained until packaging with either a vacuum mattress or a scoop stretcher, head blocks and tape is achieved.

The child's head may have to be moved to achieve a neutral in-line position as this is preferable to transporting the child with the head in an angulated position. Any attempt to move the child's head into an in-line position should be stopped if:

- There is resistance to movement
- Movement causes pain
- Any increased neurological deficit is observed

When manually immobilising the head, remember not to cover the patient's ears with your hands. Covering the ears reduces communication with the child and may frighten him or her.

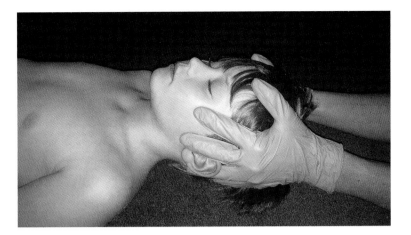

Figure 17.4 Manual in-line stabilisation

It must be remembered that, particularly under the age of 12 months, children have large occiputs. This means the neck has a tendency to flex. A small pad under the shoulders will help to maintain the head in the neutral position.

If in-line immobilisation is not possible, manual immobilisation will have to be maintained in the position found and the child immobilised using improvised equipment such as towels and blankets.

17.4 Pre-hospital immobilisation equipment

There is a wide range of equipment specifically designed for spinal immobilisation (Figure 17.5) and its use should be encouraged whenever indicated. It is the pre-hospital clinician's responsibility to choose the most appropriate immobilisation equipment available. If specialised immobilisation equipment is not available or appropriate for the given circumstance, improvisation will be required. Remember that in very young children, using the parent as a human splint will often provide a higher degree of immobilisation than many commercial devices. Caution must be taken with the transportation of the parent if this technique is chosen.

(a)

(b)

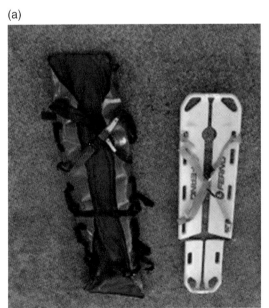
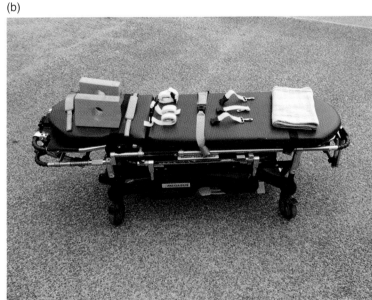

Figure 17.5 Equipment for immobilisation

Exceptions to the rule

Both the frightened, uncooperative casualty and the casualty who is hypoxic and combative may have increased cervical spine movement if padding and tape are applied. This is because these casualties may fight to escape from any restraint. In such cases manual in-line stabilisation should be maintained if tolerated, otherwise allow the child to calm down and position themselves.

Transferring a child with a suspected spinal injury from the scene of an incident to hospital requires considered and careful handling. Stages of movement should be reduced to the absolute minimum and, if possible, the single movement principle applied. There will be occasions where a child has to be rescued from a scene using an extrication device, before being transferred to an immobilisation device. Wherever possible, the child should be moved and immobilised using the same piece of equipment.

Scoop stretcher

Scoop stretchers shoud be carried as standard (Figure 17.6). The device can be split and thus applied to either side of the patient before being rejoined – thus avoiding the need for a full log roll. Only a minimal tilt is required, sufficient to allow insertion of the blades under the child. A child can be secured and transferred to hospital on the scoop stretcher, which minimises both transfer movements and on-scene time. Where a journey to hospital is expected to exceed 45 minutes, a non-time-critical child can be transferred onto a vacuum mattress, thus avoiding pressure tissue injuries.

By working to the single movement principle, any child immobilised onto a scoop stretcher should have clothing removed, thus avoiding unnecessary handling at definitive care. This 'scoop-to-skin' approach should obviously be modified to recognise environmental and dignity issues in the pre-hospital environment.

Attention should be paid to ensuring the head blocks and straps provide adequate immobilisation, as commercially available blocks and straps are not always readily available.

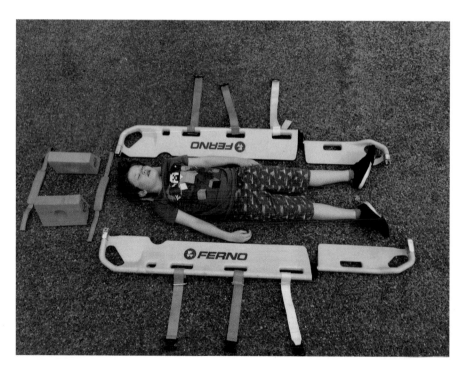

Figure 17.6 Scoop stretcher

Equipment

- Scoop stretcher
- Straps
- Blankets/padding
- Head blocks and straps/padding and tape

Procedure

1. Ensure that manual in-line cervical stabilisation is maintained by a second person throughout.
2. Explain to the child what you are going to do.
3. Adjust the stretcher to the length of the child.
4. Separate the scoop into two halves; position each half on either side of the child.
5. Position the second rescuer to one side of the child, placing one hand on the child's furthest shoulder and the other hand on the furthest pelvic crest.
6. The child should be slightly tilted towards the second rescuer – the amount of tilt should be minimised to simply allow a third rescuer to insert the blades of the scoop, but should not exceed 15°. The first rescuer who is providing manual in-line stabilisation should coordinate the movement. **The child does not need to be log rolled to insert the blades of the stretcher.**
7. The second rescuer should move to the other side of the child, and the process is repeated to insert the other half of the scoop.
8. Great care should be taken in joining both halves together. The head end should be secured first, followed by the foot end. Beware of 'pinching' the patient between both halves when connecting, particularly as the patient should be 'skin to scoop'.
9. Secure the child to the device, using three straps positioned at the child's chest, pelvis and knees. It is important to use blankets and padding in the natural hollows of the patient's contour. **Always secure the body straps first, starting with the chest and working downwards.**
10. Secure the child's head. It is likely that the equipment will need improvising to secure adequately to the scoop. It may be necessary to place the head blocks in at a different angle, thus it is essential to ensure that the head is securely immobilised.
11. Transferring the child off a scoop stretcher is the reverse of the above procedure.

Application of head blocks and straps or padding and tape

Equipment

- Head blocks and straps (commercial style)
- Blankets and tape (improvised style)

Procedure

1. Ensure that manual in-line cervical stabilisation is maintained by a second person throughout.
2. Ensure all body straps are secured first.
3. Place head blocks or blanket/pads on either side of the head at the same time.
4. Apply the forehead strap (or tape) and securely attach it to the immobilisation device. It is essential that both ends of the strap are secured at the same time, thus avoiding head movement.
5. Apply the lower strap directly over the chin and secure both ends to the immobilisation device at the same time (Figure 17.7).

Sandbags are sometimes used in hospital for head immobilisation. In the pre-hospital setting these should be avoided as they produce too many forces on the neck during transportation. Use the methods described previously.

In all cases, the pre-hospital provider should bear in mind that the decision to immobilise with full spinal protection must be justifiable. Head blocks and other immobilisation may cause extreme distress; full spinal immobilisation increases the risk of aspiration as the child will not be able to protect the airway by allowing significant fluid volumes to be expelled.

Vacuum mattress

Vacuum mattresses provide a comfortable and bespoke immobilisation platform for transporting children to hospital. Less padding is required to enable good immobilisation; however, the reliability of these devices is often called into question – usually through punctures to the material. Vacuum mattresses are not as widely available as scoop stretchers or long spinal boards. They do, however, provide a very high degree of immobilisation and patient comfort, as well being associated with the lowest incidence of pressure tissue injury. Most older children can be immobilised in an adult vacuum

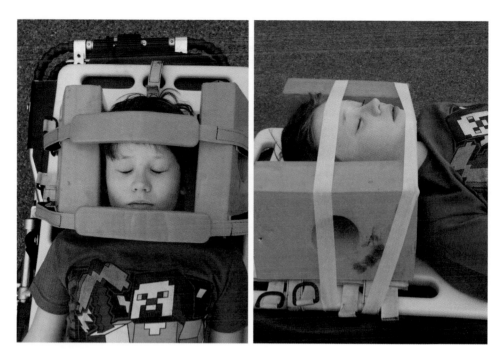

Figure 17.7 Head blocks and tape

mattress with minimal improvisation required; an adult long leg vacuum splint can also be used for smaller children and provide similar levels of comfort and immobilisation.

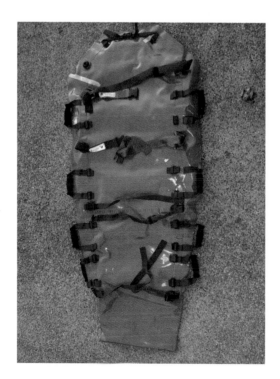

Figure 17.8 Vacuum mattress

Minimum equipment

- Vacuum mattress with straps
- Straps
- Blankets/padding

Procedure

1. Ensure that manual in-line cervical stabilisation is maintained by a second person throughout.
2. Explain to the child what you are going to do.
3. Ensure any sharp items or debris that may damage the mattress are removed.
4. Scoop the child as described previously.
5. Move the child to the centre of the vacuum mattress and place onto a draw-sheet or a patient handling sheet.
6. Remove the scoop stretcher as described previously. Ensure a rescuer maintains in-line stabilisation whilst the scoop is being removed, and continues whilst the vacuum mattress is being applied.
7. Lift the edges of the mattress and conform around the contour of the child. Shape the mattress around the head, ensuring all voids are filled and the head is sufficiently supported. Gently tightening the straps fitted to the mattress will help keep the edges in place until the device becomes rigid.
8. Evacuate the air from the vacuum mattress using the supplied vacuum pump until it becomes rigid (Figure 17.9).
9. Reassess and adjust the straps to ensure the child is secure; pay particular attention to the head and ensure it is suitably immobilised, using medical grade adhesive tape.

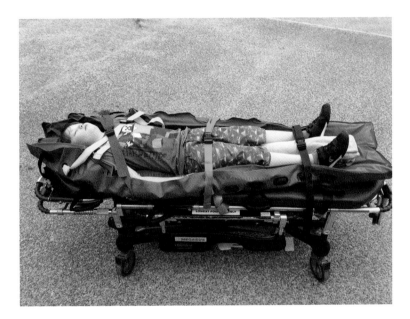

Figure 17.9 Vacuum mattress in use

Pelvic splints

Stabilisation of a pelvic injury before uncompensatable haemorrhage has occurred and clotting mechanisms are still intact should be done as early as possible after the injury. A pelvic splint should thus be applied during the circulatory element of primary survey.

When assessing a child in a trauma situation, the pelvis should not be palpated for instability or pain. A conscious child may be able to give information about pain in the lower back, groin or hips. Once a splint has been applied, analgesia may be provided to a haemodynamically stable child prior to transfer.

Procedure

1. Where possible use a splint applicator to reduce friction and patient movement.
2. Slide the pelvic splint under the patient at the level of the greater trochanters.
3. Once in place, remove the upper applicator in the same direction that it was inserted.
4. Cut away clothing to enable 'splint to skin'.
5. Ensure the splint is still located at the greater trochanter level, then fasten as per manufacturer's directions (Figure 17.10).

(a)   (b)

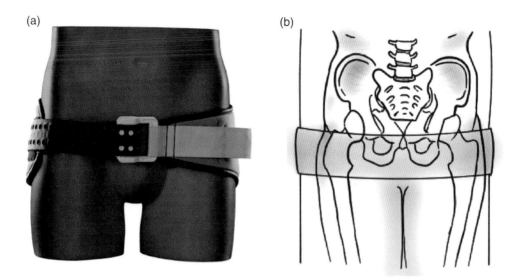

Figure 17.10 (a) SAM Pelvic Sling II. Reproduced with permission of SAM Medical. **(b) Splint near the greater trochanter.**
Adapted, with permission, of the Royal Children's Hospital, Melbourne, Australia www.rch.org.au/clinicalguide

Long spinal boards and rescue boards

Spinal boards are no longer recommended as an imobilisation device. They are still carried by many organisations but should only be used as an extrication or rescue device. If a patient has been extricated on a long board, they should be removed from this device by a scoop stretcher.

Helmet removal

Cycle or motorcycle helmets must be removed without causing cervical spine movements. This requires a minimum of two people.

1. Obtain a history of the mechanism of injury.
2. Explain the procedure to the patient and parent(s).
3. Perform a mini-neurological examination.
4. The first rescuer provides in-line immobilisation by kneeling behind the patient's head and holding the lower edge of the crash helmet on either side with each hand.
5. The second rescuer opens the face shield (removes spectacles) and undoes or cuts the chin strap, before grasping the occipital ridge with one hand and placing the thumb and forefinger of the other hand along the mandible (Figure 17.11).

(a)   (b)

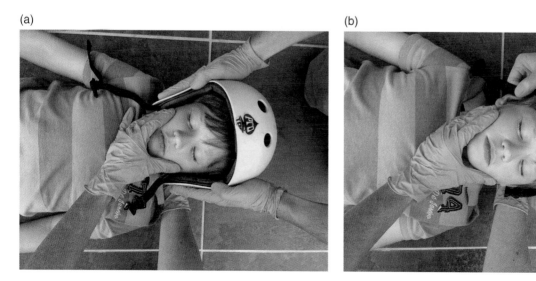

Figure 17.11 Removal of a helmet

6. The first rescuer then rotates the helmet towards himself or herself until the face bar contacts with the patient's nose and then rotates the helmet forward to clear over the patient's occiput. It may be necessary to loosen the helmet by gently pulling the sides outwards.
7. It may require further lifts of the face bar to clear the nose and then the forehead.
8. Remove the helmet over the front of the head.
9. The patient should then be secured to an immobilisation device by body straps and head blocks with head straps or tape.
10. Carry out a brief neurological examination again.

A restless, agitated child should not be fully immobilised in order to avoid inducing further cervical spine damage.

Child car seats

If a stable child is found to still be in their car seat, it may be possible to assess and transfer them to hospital in that device. Caution should be applied where the seat shows evidence of damage or where the seat cannot be properly secured within the pre-hospital vehicle.

Log rolling

In order to minimise the chances of exacerbating unrecognised spinal cord injury, non-essential movements of the spine must be avoided. If manoeuvres that might cause spinal movement are essential, for example during examination of the back during the secondary survey, then log rolling may be performed (Figure 17.12). The use of log rolling in order to place a child on an immobilisation device is no longer recommended.

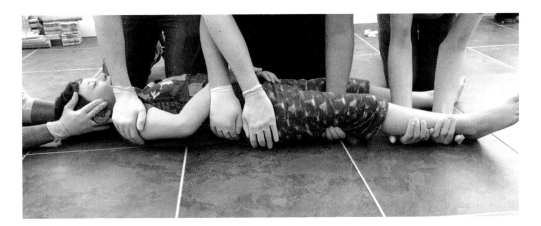

Figure 17.12 Log rolling

CHAPTER 18
Military pre-hospital paediatric care

Learning outcomes

After reading this chapter, you will be able to:
• Describe some key challenges and differences when dealing with children in the deployed military setting

18.1 Introduction

Paediatric patients have presented to military medical facilities on almost all deployments, and it is to be expected that they will continue to do so. In most cases there will be little or no specialist paediatric support available to military pre-hospital personnel; in the pre-hospital setting, you will be the paediatrician. Deploying personnel should be aware of this expectation, the different requirements of paediatric patients in the deployed medical setting and the impact they can have. As discussed previously in this manual, much of the anxiety felt when dealing with children is unnecessary. Military personnel can be encouraged by the fact that their knowledge and skill gained from training and previous operational experience will be transferrable to children and that military protocols and algorithms can be applied directly to children.

18.2 Children in the developing world

There is a far higher mortality rate in the developing world; in some areas the under 5 mortality rate is in excess of 200 per 100 000 live births compared with 40 per 100 000 in the UK. After the first month of life when prematurity is the leading single cause, diarrhoea and pneumonia account for half of all deaths. Around 7% of deaths are caused by injuries.

The contributing factors in this are:

• Water and sanitation
• Nutrition
• Infectious disease
• Safety standards
• Access to health and maternity care

Pre-Hospital Paediatric Life Support: A Practical Approach to Emergencies, Third Edition. Edited by Alan Charters, Hal Maxwell and Paul Reavley.
© 2017 John Wiley & Sons Ltd. Published 2017 by John Wiley & Sons Ltd.

Military medical personnel should be aware of the range of infectious diseases present in any given theatre. Local populations may be unvaccinated and therefore children may present with illness that is uncommonly or never seen in developed nations. These include:

- Malaria
- Tuberculosis
- Diphtheria
- Tetanus
- Polio
- Typhoid
- Parasitic infestations

18.3 Preparation for deployment

The nature of the operation will determine the likelihood of the requirement to treat children, ranging from none at all to a certainty such as in humanitarian activity. Medical planning will be based on the mission and medical intelligence. If paediatric patients are to be expected then training, equipment, personal appraisal and unit level validation should take this into account. Commanders should expect their service people to be more anxious about treating children than other patients and be aware of the negative impact of real or perceived failure on unit morale and effectiveness as well as the risk of reputational damage. Much of this can be mitigated with adequate preparation.

Personal preparation should be appropriate to role. Healthcare professionals have a duty to ensure that they are able to deliver within their scope of practice. Pre-deployment packages will provide some mission-specific training but only the individual will be aware of their own ability to deal with children. Personnel should ensure they access the correct training packages, of which military PHPLS is one, and that they have the correct clinical exposure to paediatric practice. In addition to clinical skills and knowledge, military personnel should have a full understanding of the lay down of medical assets in their theatre of operation, location and capability. This includes other troop-contributing nations, non-government organisations (NGOs) and host nation facilities.

18.4 Eligibility

On every military deployment, medical rules of eligibility (MRoE) will determine whether or not children will be able to access care at military medical facilities. On humanitarian operations this may be relatively open, however if on more offensive operations the access may be much more restricted. The primary role of military medical services is to provide medical support in order to achieve operational success. In combat the priority will be the military population at risk. This will result in difficult decisions regarding access to care for civilians, including children, so that capacity and capability are maintained.

Healthcare professionals at Role 1 locations are not expected to make these decisions in isolation and are still required to provide life-, sight and limb-saving treatment where required. Should a child present and be treated at Role 1 it will be down to the discretion of local command to provide assistance, but this decision will probably be devolved to the medical officer or senior medical and nursing staff. The medical chain of command will provide support and guide any subsequent decisions regarding rearward evacuation to Role 2 or Role 3. All children that may require rearward evacuation should be highlighted to the chain of command as soon as possible.

Children may present for non-urgent care. In these circumstances it is reasonable to direct patients to host nation or NGO facilities. The exception would be if military personnel have been directed to provide non-urgent care.

18.5 Equipment

Paediatric equipment in medical modules can be limited and is generally based on an estimate of the proportion of patients who will be children. Contemporary literature from conflicts in Afghanistan and Iraq describe a paediatric patient workload of 4–7% of patients. However, these patients had a bigger impact on resources when compared with military patients, accounting for up to 20% of intensive treatment unit bed days, longer admissions and more procedures required. If the military and medical planning process identifies a higher paediatric work load than standard doctrine assumes, equipment holdings will need to be increased. Whatever paediatric equipment and material is held, be familiar with what you hold, how to use it and capability limitations.

18.6 Military trauma in children

It is inevitable that children will become involved in conflict and will suffer military trauma. The key point is that children sustain largely the same injuries as adults, potentially in a slightly different pattern but nonetheless the same. Military personnel are trained to assess and treat trauma using the military trauma life support systems. When assessing children for injury use exactly the same system, considering the key differences that are taught on paediatric life support courses. The interventions required for life-threatening injuries are largely the same too. The military PHPLS course will further build on military trauma systems to adapt your practice to children.

18.7 Massive transfusion

Most Role 1 locations do not hold blood products. It is, however, routinely carried by advanced pre-hospital care teams such as the UK Medical Emergency Response Team. Where they are held, blood products should be administered in line with the military paediatric massive transfusion policy. As in adult populations, trauma patients requiring volume should receive blood products, not crystalloid, as the first fluids given. In summary:

- In the first hour post injury, resuscitate to a palpable radial pulse in children, and brachial in infants
- All blood products are given in 5 ml/kg boluses in a 1:1 ratio
- Tranexamic acid is to be given at 15 mg/kg to a maximum of 1 g
- 10% calcium chloride is to be given at 0.2 ml/kg to a maximum of 10 ml
- Following the first hour, fully resuscitate to normal perfusion

18.8 Medical evacuation and discharge

Disposal options from Role 1 are:

- Home
- Host nation facilities
- NGO facilities
- Role 2 or 3

It is preferable to use appropriate local or NGO facilities rather than rearward movement to military facilities. A good understanding of the lay down of medical assets, their capability and how to access them is required.

Requests for evacuation to Role 2 or 3 should be passed up the chain of command in the usual manner. The ability of Role 2 or 3 to receive children will vary with capacity, operational tempo and the MRoE.

18.9 Ethical decision making

Occasionally, it will not be possible to save a child. Very difficult decisions have to be made in the best interest of patients and sometimes on-going care will be deemed inappropriate. A good example of this is large burns that in a developed healthcare system would be treated. In a resource-limited environment where the expertise to care for complex burns patients does not exist, large burns have no possibility of a successful outcome. It therefore may be decided not to start treatment but to provide end of life care only. This is exceptionally difficult to deal with, but represents the reality of the environments in which military personnel are occasionally required to operate. Personnel should be prepared for decisions such as this. Role 1 personnel are not expected to routinely make these decisions; advice should be sought from the medical chain of command.

18.10 Safeguarding

Different cultures have different approaches to safeguarding, from a developed world perspective social care and child protection may appear inadequate or even non-existent in some nations. Military personnel still have an absolute responsibility to protect a child from harm while that child is in the care of the Defence Medical Services and to do all they can to prevent further harm on discharge. Children should always be accompanied by parents or guardians. However, if there are security risks associated with allowing accompanying adults access to military locations, then safety is the priority. If a child is moved rearward without accompanying guardians then it is vital that the identity of the child and their parents/guardians is established in order to ensure safe subsequent discharge.

18.11 Resources (UK military)

Military paediatric guidance is available in the UK Ministry of Defence *Clinical Guidelines for Operations* (CGO) (https://www.gov.uk/government/publications/jsp-999-clinical-guidelines-for-operations, last accessed March 2017). This is an open source document. Additionally, guidelines pending publication in CGOs are held on the Defence Gateway Anaesthetic and Deployed Paediatric Special Interest Group pages (https://sts.defencegateway.mod.uk/register.aspx last accessed March 2017).

Advice on policy, manning, equipment, training and clinical guidance can be obtained from the Deployed Paediatric Special Interest Group, contacted by emailing: depsig.mod@nhs.net

APPENDIX
Paediatric emergency reference cards

The cards reproduced in this appendix are an example of a rapid reference tool for paediatric pre-hospital emergency care also known as a 'page per age reference tool'. This set belongs to the Great Western Air Ambulance, Bristol, UK. Each pair of cards provides estimated weight for age, normal ranges for vital observations (based on the 50th centile), and reference doses for equipment, drugs and therapies commonly used by the team when caring for critically unwell children. The designs are modified, by permission, from those used by Sydney Helicopter Emergency Medical Service (HEMS), originally designed by Karol Habig and Chris Hill, and are correct at the time of publishing (for updates see www.alsg.org).

Great Western Air Ambulance is a charitably funded air ambulance charity founded in 2007. Its teams of critical care specialist paramedics and HEMS physicians respond as part of Southwest Ambulance Service NHS Foundation Trust, delivering the complete range of pre-hospital critical care interventions to patients of all ages across a population of 2.3 million inhabitants in the southwest of the UK. They average 4.6 call-outs per day, of which approximately 10% are children under the age of 16 with critical illness or major trauma.

Abbreviations used in the appendix	
BP	blood pressure
BVM	bag–valve–mask
ETT	endotracheal tube
GCS	Glasgow Coma Scale
HR	heart rate
IM	intramuscular
IV	intravenous
mcg	micrograms
PHEA	pre-hospital emergency anaesthesia
RR	respiratory rate
SOP	standard operating procedure
SVT	supraventricular tachycardia
TXA	tranexamic acid

Pre-Hospital Paediatric Life Support: A Practical Approach to Emergencies, Third Edition. Edited by Alan Charters, Hal Maxwell and Paul Reavley.
© 2017 John Wiley & Sons Ltd. Published 2017 by John Wiley & Sons Ltd.

PAEDIATRIC
EMERGENCY
REFERENCE CARDS

Quick Reference for Paediatric Patients

Age Specific Pages include:
PHEA essentials
Critical Care Reference
Paediatric Forumulary

FOR GUIDANCE ONLY
Please use individual clinical judgement

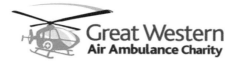
Great Western
Air Ambulance Charity

Weight estimates are taken from APLS 6e. If you know actual (recent) weight or your patient appears large or small for age, please use an appropriate card to avoid over or under dosage.

Ensure familiarity with equipment and always follow unit standard operating procedures.

Defibrillation energies state dare correct for Zoll X-Series monitor/defibrillator.

Refer to intranasal medications SOP for management of dead space prior to preparing or administering any intranasal medications.

When reconstituting any medication, refer to the recommended concentration stated in this resource and check prior to administration.

These cards are intended as a guide for the management of paediatric emergencies. All clinicians should exercise clinical judgement in their practice.

If you notice problems or have feedback please email the authors at the earliest opportunity:

jim.blackburn@doctors.net.uk
&
james.tooley@nhs.net

Preterm 23 weeks – 0.5 kg

NORMAL VITAL SIGNS

RR	Tidal vol.	HR	Sys. BP
40–60	BVM ± 3 ml	120–160	>32 mmHg

FLUID BOLUS

5 ml/kg	10 ml/kg	20 ml/kg	Blood – 5 ml/kg
2.5 ml	5 ml	10 ml	2.5 ml

AIRWAY

ETT size	ETT length	Laryngoscopy	Miller 0
2.5 uncuffed	6.5 cm	Bougie = 6 Ch (neonatal)	i-gel = n/a

PRE-HOSPITAL EMERGENCY ANAESTHESIA

Fentanyl	3 mcg/kg 50 mcg/ml	1.5 mcg	0.03 ml
Ketamine	Not used in preterms		
Rocuronium	1 mg/kg 10 mg/ml	0.5 mg	0.05 ml

SEDATION

Morphine	0.1 mg/kg 1 mg/ml	0.05 mg	0.05 ml
Midazolam	0.1 mg/kg 1 mg/ml	0.05 mg	0.05 ml
Ketamine	Not used in preterms		

Preterm 23 weeks – 0.5 kg

Preterm 23 weeks – 0.5 kg

FLUID – OTHER

Glucose 10%		2.5 ml/kg	1.3 ml
Hypertonic saline		3 ml/kg	n/a

CARDIOVASCULAR

Defibrillation 4 J/kg	Arrest	–	–
Adrenaline 1:10000 10 mcg/kg	Arrest	5 mcg	0.05 ml
Amiodarone 5 mg/kg (30 mg/ml)	Arrest	2.5 mg	0.08 ml
Sodium bicarb. (8.4%)	Arrest/cardiac	0.5 mmol	0.5 ml
Calcium chloride (10%)	Cardiac/blood	–	0.05 ml
Adrenaline 1:100000 0.15 mcg/kg	Inotrope	0.08 mcg	0.01 ml
Adrenaline 1:1000 10 mcg/kg	Anaphylaxis	5 mcg IM	0.005 ml
Adrenaline 1:100000 1 mcg/kg	Anaphylaxis	0.5 mcg IV	0.05 ml (1:100 000)
Atropine 20 mcg/kg (600 mcg/ml)	HR 60	10 mcg	0.02 ml
Adenosine 150 mcg/kg (3 mg/ml)	SVT	0.08 mg	0.03 ml

OTHER

Ceftriaxone 50 mg/kg (100 mg/ml)	Sepsis	25 mg	0.25 ml
Diazepam IV 0.4 mg/kg (10 mg/ml)	Seizure	0.2 mg (max. 2 doses)	0.02 ml (max. 2 doses)
Nasal fentanyl 1.5 mcg/kg (50 mcg/ml)	NOT USED IN PRETERMS		
TXA 15 mg/kg (100 mg/ml)	Trauma	7.5 mg	0.08 ml

Preterm 23 weeks – 0.5 kg

Preterm 27 weeks – 1 kg

NORMAL VITAL SIGNS

RR	HR	Sys. BP
40–60	120–160	>40 mmHg

FLUID BOLUS

5 ml/kg	10 ml/kg	Blood – 5 ml/kg
5 ml	10 ml	5 ml

AIRWAY

ETT size	ETT length	Laryngoscopy
3 uncuffed	7 cm	Miller 0

Bougie = 6 Ch (neonatal)
i-gel = n/a

PRE-HOSPITAL EMERGENCY ANAESTHESIA

Fentanyl	3 mcg/kg	3 mcg	0.06 ml
	50 mcg/ml		
Ketamine	Not used in preterms		
Rocuronium	1 mg/kg	1 mg	0.1 ml
	10 mg/ml		

SEDATION

Morphine	0.1 mg/kg	0.1 mg	0.1 ml
	1 mg/ml		
Midazolam	0.1 mg/kg	0.1 mg	0.1 ml
	1 mg/ml		
Ketamine	Not used in preterms		

Preterm 27 weeks – 1 kg

FLUID – OTHER

Glucose 10%	2.5 ml/kg	2.5 ml
Hypertonic saline	3 ml/kg	n/a

CARDIOVASCULAR

Defibrillation 4 J/kg		5 J	2.5 ml
Adrenaline 1:10 000 10 mcg/kg	Arrest	10 mcg	0.1 ml
Amiodarone 5 mg/kg (30 mg/ml)	Arrest	5 mg	0.17 ml
Sodium bicarb. (8.4%)	Arrest/cardiac	1 mmol	1 ml
Calcium chloride (10%)	Cardiac/blood	–	0.1 ml
Adrenaline 1:100 000 0.15 mcg/kg	Inotrope	0.15 mcg	0.02 ml
Adrenaline 1:1000 10 mcg/kg	Anaphylaxis	10 mcg IM	0.01 ml
Adrenaline 1:100 000 1 mcg/kg	Anaphylaxis	1 mcg IV	0.1 ml (1:100 000)
Atropine 20 mcg/kg (600 mcg/ml)	HR 60	20 mcg	0.03 ml
Adenosine 150 mcg/kg (3 mg/ml)	SVT	0.15 mg	0.05 ml

OTHER

Ceftriaxone 50 mg/kg (100 mg/ml)	Sepsis	50 mg	0.5 ml
Diazepam IV 0.4 mg/kg (10 mg/ml)	Seizure	0.4 mg (max. 2 doses)	0.04 ml (max. 2 doses)
Nasal fentanyl 1.5 mcg/kg (50 mcg/ml)	NOT USED IN PRETERMS		
TXA 15 mg/kg (100 mg/ml)	Trauma	15 mg	0.15 ml

Preterm 33 weeks – 2 kg

NORMAL VITAL SIGNS

RR	Tidal vol.	HR	Sys. BP
40–60	BVM ± 12 ml	120–160	>40 mmHg

FLUID BOLUS

5 ml/kg	20 ml/kg	Blood – 5 ml/kg
10 ml	40 ml	10 ml

AIRWAY

ETT size	ETT length	Laryngoscopy	Miller 0/1
3 uncuffed	8 cm	Bougie = 6 Ch (neonatal)	
		i-gel = 1 (pink)	

PRE-HOSPITAL EMERGENCY ANAESTHESIA

Fentanyl	3 mcg/kg	6 mcg	50 mcg/ml	0.12 ml
Ketamine	Not used in preterms			
Rocuronium	1 mg/kg	2 mg	10 mg/ml	0.2 ml

SEDATION

Morphine	0.1 mg/kg	0.2 mg	1 mg/ml	0.2 ml
Midazolam	0.1 mg/kg	0.2 mg	1 mg/ml	0.2 ml
Ketamine	Not used in preterms			

Preterm 33 weeks – 2 kg

Preterm 33 weeks – 2 kg

FLUID – OTHER

Glucose 10%	2.5 ml/kg	5 ml
Hypertonic saline	3 ml/kg	n/a

CARDIOVASCULAR

Defibrillation 4 J/kg		10 J	
Adrenaline 1:10 000 10 mcg/kg	Arrest	20 mcg	0.2 ml
Amiodarone 5 mg/kg (30 mg/ml)	Arrest	10 mg	0.33 ml
Sodium bicarb. (8.4%)	Arrest/cardiac	2 mmol	2 ml
Calcium chloride (10%)	Cardiac/blood	–	0.2 ml
Adrenaline 1:100 000 0.15 mcg/kg	Inotrope	0.3 mcg	0.03 ml
Adrenaline 1:1000 10 mcg/kg	Anaphylaxis	20 mcg IM	0.02 ml
Adrenaline 1:100 000 1 mcg/kg	Anaphylaxis	2 mcg IV	0.2 ml (1:100 000)
Atropine 20 mcg/kg (600 mcg/ml)	HR 60	40 mcg	0.07 ml
Adenosine 150 mcg/kg (3 mg/ml)	SVT	0.3 mg	0.1 ml

OTHER

Ceftriaxone 50 mg/kg (100 mg/ml)	Sepsis	100 mg	1 ml
Diazepam IV 0.4 mg/kg (10 mg/ml)	Seizure	0.8 mg (max. 2 doses)	0.08 ml (max. 2 doses)
Nasal fentanyl 1.5 mcg/kg (50 mcg/ml)	NOT USED IN PRETERMS		
TXA 15 mg/kg (100 mg/ml)	Trauma	30 mg	0.3 ml

Preterm 33 weeks – 2 kg

Newborn (term) – 3.5 kg

NORMAL VITAL SIGNS

RR	Tidal vol.	HR	Sys. BP
25–50	BVM ±20 ml	120–170	>70 mmHg

FLUID BOLUS

5 ml/kg	10 ml/kg	20 ml/kg	Blood – 5 ml/kg
17.5 ml	35 ml	70 ml	17.5 ml

AIRWAY

ETT size	ETT length	Laryngoscopy	
3.5 cuffed	9.5 cm	Miller 1	Bougie = 6 Ch (neonatal) i-gel = 1 (pink)

PRE-HOSPITAL EMERGENCY ANAESTHESIA

Drug	Dose		
Fentanyl	3 mcg/kg 50 mcg/ml	10.5 mcg	0.21 ml
Ketamine	2 mg/kg 10 mg/ml	7 mg	0.7 ml
Rocuronium	1 mg/kg 10 mg/ml	3.5 mg	0.35 ml

SEDATION

Drug	Dose		
Morphine	0.1 mg/kg 1 mg/ml	0.35 mg	0.35 ml
Midazolam	0.1 mg/kg 1 mg/ml	0.35 mg	0.35 ml
Ketamine	0.5 mg/kg 10 mg/ml	1.75 mg	0.18 ml

Newborn (term) – 3.5 kg

FLUID – OTHER

Glucose 10%	2.5 ml/kg	8.8 ml
Hypertonic saline	3 ml/kg	10.5 ml

CARDIOVASCULAR

Drug	Indication	Dose	Volume
Defibrillation 4 J/kg	Arrest	15 J	
Adrenaline 1:10 000 10 mcg/kg	Arrest	35 mcg	0.35 ml
Amiodarone 5 mg/kg (30 mg/ml)	Arrest	17.5 mg	0.58 ml
Sodium bicarb. (8.4%)	Arrest/cardiac	3.5 mmol	3.5 ml
Calcium chloride (10%)	Cardiac/blood	–	0.35 ml
Adrenaline 1:100 000 0.15 mcg/kg	Inotrope	0.53 mcg	0.05 ml
Adrenaline 1:1000 10 mcg/kg	Anaphylaxis	35 mcg IM	0.035 ml
Adrenaline 1:100 000 1 mcg/kg	Anaphylaxis	3.5 mcg IV	0.35 ml (1:100 000)
Atropine 20 mcg/kg (600 mcg/ml)	HR 60	70 mcg	0.12 ml
Adenosine 150 mcg/kg (3 mg/ml)	SVT	0.525 mg	0.18 ml

OTHER

Drug	Indication	Dose	Volume
Ceftriaxone 50 mg/kg (100 mg/ml)	Sepsis	175 mg	1.75 ml
Diazepam IV 0.4 mg/kg (10 mg/ml)	Seizure	1.4 mg (max. 2 doses)	0.14 ml (max. 2 doses)
Nasal fentanyl 1.5 mcg/kg (50 mcg/ml)	NOT USED IN NEONATES		
TXA 15 mg/kg (100 mg/ml)	Trauma	52.5 mg	0.53 ml

Newborn (term) – 3.5 kg

1 month – 4.5 kg

NORMAL VITAL SIGNS

RR	Tidal vol.	HR	Sys. BP
25–50	BVM ± 25 ml	120–170	>70 mmHg

FLUID BOLUS

5 ml/kg	10 ml/kg	20 ml/kg	Blood – 5 ml/kg
22.5 ml	45 ml	90 ml	22.5 ml

AIRWAY

ETT size	ETT length	Laryngoscope	Miller 1
4 cuffed	10 cm	Bougie = 6 Ch (neonatal)	i-gel = 1 (pink)

PRE-HOSPITAL EMERGENCY ANAESTHESIA

Fentanyl	3 mcg/kg	13.5 mcg	0.27 ml
	50 mcg/ml		
Ketamine	2 mg/kg	9 mg	0.9 ml
	10 mg/ml		
Rocuronium	1 mg/kg	4.5 mg	0.45 ml
	10 mg/ml		

SEDATION

Morphine	0.1 mg/kg	0.45 mg	0.45 ml
	1 mg/ml		
Midazolam	0.1 mg/kg	0.45 mg	0.45 ml
	1 mg/ml		
Ketamine	0.5 mg/kg	2.25 mg	0.23 ml
	10 mg/ml		

1 month – 4.5 kg

FLUID – OTHER

Glucose 10%	2 ml/kg	9 ml
Hypertonic saline	3 ml/kg	13.5 ml

CARDIOVASCULAR

Defibrillation 4 J/kg		20 J	
Adrenaline 1:10 000 10 mcg/kg	Arrest	45 mcg	0.45 ml
Amiodarone 5 mg/kg (30 mg/ml)	Arrest	22.5 mg	0.75 ml
Sodium bicarb. (8.4%)	Arrest/cardiac	4.5 mmol	4.5 ml
Calcium chloride (10%)	Cardiac/blood	–	0.45 ml
Adrenaline 1:100 000 0.15 mcg/kg	Inotrope	0.68 mcg	0.07 ml
Adrenaline 1:1000 10 mcg/kg	Anaphylaxis	45 mcg IM	0.045 ml
Adrenaline 1:100 000 1 mcg/kg	Anaphylaxis	4.5 mcg IV	0.45 ml (1:100 000)
Atropine 20 mcg/kg (600 mcg/ml)	HR 60	90 mcg	0.15 ml
Adenosine 150 mcg/kg (3 mg/ml)	SVT	0.68 mg	0.23 ml

OTHER

Ceftriaxone 50 mg/kg (100 mg/ml)	Sepsis	225 mg	2.25 ml
Diazepam IV 0.4 mg/kg (10 mg/ml)	Seizure	1.8 mg (max. 2 doses)	0.18 ml (max. 2 doses)
Nasal fentanyl 1.5 mcg/kg (50 mcg/ml)	Analgesia	6.75 mcg	0.14 ml
TXA 15 mg/kg (100 mg/ml)	Trauma	67.5 mg	0.68 ml

1 month – 4.5 kg

3 months – 6.5 kg

FLUID – OTHER

Glucose 10%	2 ml/kg	13 ml
Hypertonic saline	3 ml/kg	19.5 ml

CARDIOVASCULAR

Defibrillation 4 J/kg		25 J	
Adrenaline 1:10 000 10 mcg/kg	Arrest	65 mcg	0.65 ml
Amiodarone 5 mg/kg (30 mg/ml)	Arrest	32.5 mg	1.08 ml
Sodium bicarb. (8.4%)	Arrest/cardiac	6.5 mmol	6.5 ml
Calcium chloride (10%)	Cardiac/blood	–	0.65 ml
Adrenaline 1:100 000 0.15 mcg/kg	Inotrope	0.98 mcg	0.1 ml
Adrenaline 1:1000 10 mcg/kg	Anaphylaxis	65 mcg IM	0.065 ml
Adrenaline 1:100 000 1 mcg/kg	Anaphylaxis	6.5 mcg IV	0.65 ml (1:100 000)
Atropine 20 mcg/kg (600 mcg/ml)	HR 60	130 mcg	0.22 ml
Adenosine 150 mcg/kg (3 mg/ml)	SVT	0.98 mg	0.33 ml

OTHER

Cefotaxime 50 mg/kg (100 mg/ml)	Sepsis	325 mg	3.25 ml
Diazepam IV 0.4 mg/kg (10 mg/ml)	Seizure	2.6 mg (max. 2 doses)	0.26 ml (max. 2 doses)
Nasal fentanyl 1.5 mcg/kg (50 mcg/ml)	Analgesia	9.75 mcg	0.2 ml
TXA 15 mg/kg (100 mg/ml)	Trauma	97.5 mg	0.98 ml

3 months – 6.5 kg

NORMAL VITAL SIGNS

RR	Tidal vol.	HR	Sys. BP
25–45	BVM ± 35 ml	115–160	>70 mmHg

FLUID BOLUS

5 ml/kg	10 ml/kg	20 ml/kg	Blood – 5 ml/kg
32.5 ml	65 ml	130 ml	32.5 ml

AIRWAY

ETT size	ETT length	Laryngoscopy	Miller 1
4 cuffed	11.5 cm	Bougie = 6 Ch (neonatal)	i-gel = 1.5 (blue)

PRE-HOSPITAL EMERGENCY ANAESTHESIA

Fentanyl	3 mcg/kg / 50 mcg/ml	19.5 mcg	0.39 ml
Ketamine	2 mg/kg / 10 mg/ml	13 mg	1.3 ml
Rocuronium	1 mg/kg / 10 mg/ml	6.5 mg	0.65 ml

SEDATION

Morphine	0.1 mg/kg / 1 mg/ml	0.65 mg	0.65 ml
Midazolam	0.1 mg/kg / 1 mg/ml	0.65 mg	0.65 ml
Ketamine	0.5 mg/kg / 10 mg/ml	3.25 mg	0.33 ml

3 months – 6.5 kg

NORMAL VITAL SIGNS

RR	Tidal vol.	HR	Sys. BP
20–40	48 ml	110–160	>75 mmHg

FLUID BOLUS

			Blood – 5 ml/kg
5 ml/kg	10 ml/kg	20 ml/kg	
40 ml	80 ml	160 ml	40 ml

AIRWAY

ETT size	ETT length	Laryngoscopy
4 cuffed	12 cm	Miller 1

Bougie = 6 Ch (neonatal)
i-gel = 1.5 (blue)

PRE-HOSPITAL EMERGENCY ANAESTHESIA

Fentanyl	3 mcg/kg 50 mcg/ml	24 mcg	0.48 ml
Ketamine	2 mg/kg 10 mg/ml	16 mg	1.6 ml
Rocuronium	1 mg/kg 10 mg/ml	8 mg	0.8 ml

SEDATION

Morphine	0.1 mg/kg 1 mg/ml	0.8 mg	0.8 ml
Midazolam	0.1 mg/kg 1 mg/ml	0.8 mg	0.8 ml
Ketamine	0.5 mg/kg 10 mg/ml	4 mg	0.4 ml

FLUID – OTHER

Glucose 10%	2 ml/kg	16 ml
Hypertonic saline	3 ml/kg	24 ml

CARDIOVASCULAR

Defibrillation	4 J/kg	30 J	
Adrenaline 1:10 000 10 mcg/kg	Arrest	80 mcg	0.8 ml
Amiodarone 5 mg/kg (30 mg/ml)	Arrest	40 mg	1.33 ml
Sodium bicarb. (8.4%)	Arrest/cardiac	8 mmol	8 ml
Calcium chloride (10%)	Cardiac/blood	–	0.8 ml
Adrenaline 1:100 000 0.15 mcg/kg	Inotrope	1.2 mcg	0.12 ml
Adrenaline 1:1000 10 mcg/kg	Anaphylaxis	80 mcg IM	0.08 ml
Adrenaline 1:100 000 1 mcg/kg	Anaphylaxis	8 mcg IV	0.8 ml (1:100 000)
Atropine 20 mcg/kg (600 mcg/ml)	HR 60	160 mcg	0.27 ml
Adenosine 150 mcg/kg (3 mg/ml)	SVT	1.2 mg	0.4 ml

OTHER

Cefotaxime 50 mg/kg (100 mg/ml)	Sepsis	400 mg	4 ml
Diazepam IV 0.4 mg/kg (10 mg/ml)	Seizure	3.2 mg (max. 2 doses)	0.32 ml (max. 2 doses)
Nasal fentanyl 1.5 mcg/kg (50 mcg/ml)	Analgesia	12 mcg	0.24 ml
TXA 15 mg/kg (100 mg/ml)	Trauma	120 mg	1.2 ml

1 year – 9.5 kg

NORMAL VITAL SIGNS

RR	Tidal vol.	HR	Sys. BP
20–40	57 ml	110–160	>75 mmHg

FLUID BOLUS

5 ml/kg	10 ml/kg	20 ml/kg	Blood – 5 ml/kg
47.5 ml	95 ml	190 ml	47.5 ml

AIRWAY

ETT size	ETT length	Laryngoscopy	Miller 1
4.5 cuffed	12.5 cm	Bougie = 10 Ch (paed.)	i-gel = 1.5 (blue)

PRE-HOSPITAL EMERGENCY ANAESTHESIA

Drug	Dose	Conc.		
Fentanyl	3 mcg/kg	50 mcg/ml	28.5 mcg	0.57 ml
Ketamine	2 mg/kg	10 mg/ml	19 mg	1.9 ml
Rocuronium	1 mg/kg	10 mg/ml	9.5 mg	0.95 ml

SEDATION

Drug	Dose	Conc.		
Morphine	0.1 mg/kg	1 mg/ml	0.95 mg	0.95 ml
Midazolam	0.1 mg/kg	1 mg/ml	0.95 mg	0.95 ml
Ketamine	0.5 mg/kg	10 mg/ml	4.75 mg	0.48 ml

1 year – 9.5 kg

---

1 year – 9.5 kg

FLUID – OTHER

Glucose 10%	2 ml/kg	19 ml
Hypertonic saline	3 ml/kg	28.5 ml

CARDIOVASCULAR

Drug	Indication	Dose	Volume
Defibrillation 4 J/kg	Arrest	40 J	
Adrenaline 1:10 000 10 mcg/kg	Arrest	95 mcg	0.95 ml
Amiodarone 5 mg/kg (30 mg/ml)	Arrest	47.5 mg	1.58 ml
Sodium bicarb. (8.4%)	Arrest/cardiac	9.5 mmol	9.5 ml
Calcium chloride (10%)	Cardiac/blood	–	0.95 ml
Adrenaline 1:100 000 0.15 mcg/kg	Inotrope	1.43 mcg	0.14 ml
Adrenaline 1:1000 10 mcg/kg	Anaphylaxis	95 mcg IM	0.095 ml
Adrenaline 1:100 000 1 mcg/kg	Anaphylaxis	9.5 mcg IV	0.95 ml (1:100 000)
Atropine 20 mcg/kg (600 mcg/ml)	HR 60	190 mcg	0.32 ml
Adenosine 150 mcg/kg (3 mg/ml)	SVT	1.43 mg	0.48 ml

OTHER

Drug	Indication	Dose	Volume
Cefotaxime 50 mg/kg (100 mg/ml)	Sepsis	475 mg	4.75 ml
Diazepam IV 0.4 mg/kg (10 mg/ml)	Seizure	3.8 mg (max. 2 doses)	0.38 ml (max. 2 doses)
Nasal fentanyl 1.5 mcg/kg (50 mcg/ml)	Analgesia	14.25 mcg	0.29 ml
TXA 15 mg/kg (100 mg/ml)	Trauma	142.5 mg	1.43 ml

1 year – 9.5 kg

2 years – 12 kg

NORMAL VITAL SIGNS

RR	Tidal vol.	HR	Sys. BP
20–30	72 ml	100–150	>75 mmHg

FLUID BOLUS

5 ml/kg	10 ml/kg	20 ml/kg	Blood – 5 ml/kg bolus	
60 ml	120 ml	240 ml	60 ml	

AIRWAY

ETT size	ETT length	Laryngoscope	Mac 2
4.5 cuffed	13 cm	Bougie = 10 Ch (paed.)	i-gel = 2 (grey)

PRE-HOSPITAL EMERGENCY ANAEST–ESIA

Fentanyl	3 mcg/kg / 50 mcg/ml	36 mcg	0.72 ml
Ketamine	2 mg/kg / 10 mg/ml	24 mg	2.4 ml
Rocuronium	1 mg/kg / 10 mg/ml	12 mg	1.2 ml

SEDATION

Morphine	0.1 mg/kg / 1 mg/ml	1.2 mg	1.2 ml
Midazolam	0.1 mg/kg / 1 mg/ml	1.2 mg	1.2 ml
Ketamine	0.5 mg/kg / 10 mg/ml	6 mg	0.6 ml

2 years – 12 kg

---

2 years – 12 kg

FLUID – OTHER

Glucose 10%	2 ml/kg		24 ml
Hypertonic saline	3 ml/kg		36 ml

CARDIOVASCULAR

Defibrillation 4 J/kg		50 J	
Adrenaline 1:10 000 10 mcg/kg	Arrest	120 mcg	1.2 ml
Amiodarone 5 mg/kg (30 mg/ml)	Arrest	60 mg	2 ml
Sodium bicarb. (8.4%)	Arrest/cardiac	12 mmol	12 ml
Calcium chloride (10%)	Cardiac/blood	–	1.2 ml
Adrenaline 1:100 000 0.15 mcg/kg	Inotrope	1.8 mcg	0.18 ml
Adrenaline 1:1000 10 mcg/kg	Anaphylaxis	120 mcg IM	0.12 ml
Adrenaline 1:100 000 1 mcg/kg	Anaphylaxis	12 mcg IV	1.2 ml (1:100 000)
Atropine 20 mcg/kg (600 mcg/ml)	HR 60	240 mcg	0.4 ml
Adenosine 150 mcg/kg (3 mg/ml)	SVT	1.8 mg	0.6 ml

OTHER

Cefotaxime 50 mg/kg (100 mg/ml)	Sepsis	600 mg	6 ml
Diazepam IV 0.4 mg/kg (10 mg/ml)	Seizure	4.8 mg (max. 2 doses)	0.48 ml (max. 2 doses)
Nasal fentanyl 1.5 mcg/kg (50 mcg/ml)	Analgesia	18 mcg	0.36 ml
TXA 15 mg/kg (100 mg/ml)	Trauma	180 mg	1.8 ml

2 years – 12 kg

3 years – 14 kg

NORMAL VITAL SIGNS

RR	Tidal vol.	HR	Sys. BP
20–30	84 ml	90–140	>80 mmHg

FLUID BOLUS

5 ml/kg	10 ml/kg	20 ml/kg	Blood – 5 ml/kg bolus
70 ml	140 ml	280 ml	70 ml

AIRWAY

ETT size	ETT length	Laryngoscopy	
5 cuffed	13.5 cm	Bougie = 10 Ch (paed.) i-gel = 2 (grey)	Mac 2

PRE-HOSPITAL EMERGENCY ANAESTHESIA

Fentanyl	3 mcg/kg 50 mcg/ml	42 mcg	0.84 ml
Ketamine	2 mg/kg 10 mg/ml	28 mg	2.8 ml
Rocuronium	1 mg/kg 10 mg/ml	14 mg	1.4 ml

SEDATION

Morphine	0.1 mg/kg 1 mg/ml	1.4 mg	1.4 ml
Midazolam	0.1 mg/kg 1 mg/ml	1.4 mg	1.4 ml
Ketamine	0.5 mg/kg 10 mg/ml	7 mg	0.7 ml

3 years – 14 kg

---

3 years – 14 kg

FLUID – OTHER

Glucose 10%	2 ml/kg	28 ml
Hypertonic saline	3 ml/kg	42 ml

CARDIOVASCULAR

Defibrillation 4 J/kg		55 J	
Adrenaline 1:10 000 10 mcg/kg	Arrest	140 mcg	1.4 ml
Amiodarone 5 mg/kg (30 mg/ml)	Arrest	70 mg	2.33 ml
Sodium bicarb. (8.4%)	Arrest/cardiac	14 mmol	14 ml
Calcium chloride (10%)	Cardiac/blood	–	1.4 ml
Adrenaline 1:100 000 0.15 mcg/kg	Inotrope	2.1 mcg	0.21 ml
Adrenaline 1:1000 10 mcg/kg	Anaphylaxis	140 mcg IM	0.14 ml
Adrenaline 1:100 000 1 mcg/kg	Anaphylaxis	14 mcg IV	1.4 ml (1:100 000)
Atropine 20 mcg/kg (600 mcg/ml)	HR 60	280 mcg	0.47 ml
Adenosine 150 mcg/kg (3 mg/ml)	SVT	2.1 mg	0.7 ml

OTHER

Cefotaxime 50 mg/kg (100 mg/ml)	Sepsis	700 mg	7 ml
Diazepam IV 0.4 mg/kg (10 mg/ml)	Seizure	5.6 mg (max. 2 doses)	0.56 ml (max. 2 doses)
Nasal fentanyl 1.5 mcg/kg (50 mcg/ml)	Analgesia	21 mcg	0.42 ml
TXA 15 mg/kg (100 mg/ml)	Trauma	210 mg	2.1 ml

3 years – 14 kg

4 years – 16 kg

NORMAL VITAL SIGNS

RR	Tidal vol.	HR	Sys. BP
20–30	96 ml	80–135	>85 mmHg

FLUID BOLUS

5 ml/kg	10 ml/kg	20 ml/kg	Blood – 5 ml/kg bolus
80 ml	160 ml	320 ml	80 ml

AIRWAY

ETT size	Laryngoscopy
ETT length 14 cm	Mac 2
5 cuffed	Bougie = 10 Ch (paed.)
	i-gel = 2 (grey)

PRE-HOSPITAL EMERGENCY ANAESTHESIA

Drug	Dose	Amount	Volume
Fentanyl	3 mcg/kg / 50 mcg/ml	48 mcg	0.96 ml
Ketamine	2 mg/kg / 10 mg/ml	32 mg	3.2 ml
Rocuronium	1 mg/kg / 10 mg/ml	16 mg	1.6 ml

SEDATION

Drug	Dose	Amount	Volume
Morphine	0.1 mg/kg / 1 mg/ml	1.6 mg	1.6 ml
Midazolam	0.1 mg/kg / 1 mg/ml	1.6 mg	1.6 ml
Ketamine	0.5 mg/kg / 10 mg/ml	8 mg	0.8 ml

4 years – 16 kg

FLUID – OTHER

Glucose 10%		2 ml/kg	32 ml
Hypertonic saline		3 ml/kg	48 ml

CARDIOVASCULAR

Drug	Indication	Dose	Volume
Defibrillation 4 J/kg	Arrest		65 J
Adrenaline 1:10 000 10 mcg/kg	Arrest	160 mcg	1.6 ml
Amiodarone 5 mg/kg (30 mg/ml)	Arrest	80 mg	2.67 ml
Sodium bicarb. (8.4%)	Arrest/cardiac	16 mmol	16 ml
Calcium chloride (10%)	Cardiac/blood	–	1.6 ml
Adrenaline 1:100 000 0.15 mcg/kg	Inotrope	2.4 mcg	0.24 ml
Adrenaline 1:1000 10 mcg/kg	Anaphylaxis	160 mcg IM	0.16 ml
Adrenaline 1:100 000 1 mcg/kg	Anaphylaxis	16 mcg IV	1.6 ml (1:100 000)
Atropine 20 mcg/kg (600 mcg/ml)	HR 60	320 mcg	0.53 ml
Adenosine 150 mcg/kg (3 mg/ml)	SVT	2.4 mg	0.8 ml

OTHER

Drug	Indication	Dose	Volume
Cefotaxime 50 mg/kg (100 mg/ml)	Sepsis	800 mg	8 ml
Diazepam IV 0.4 mg/kg (10 mg/ml)	Seizure	6.4 mg (max. 2 doses)	0.64 ml (max. 2 doses)
Nasal fentanyl 1.5 mcg/kg (50 mcg/ml)	Analgesia	24 mcg	0.48 ml
TXA 15 mg/kg (100 mg/ml)	Trauma	240 mg	2.4 ml

4 years – 16 kg

5 years – 18 kg

FLUID – OTHER

Glucose 10%	2 ml/kg	36 ml
Hypertonic saline	3 ml/kg	54 ml

CARDIOVASCULAR

Defibrillation 4 J/kg		70 J	
Adrenaline 1:10 000 10 mcg/kg	Arrest	180 mcg	1.8 ml
Amiodarone 5 mg/kg (30 mg/ml)	Arrest	90 mg	3 ml
Sodium bicarb. (8.4%)	Arrest/cardiac	18 mmol	18 ml
Calcium chloride (10%)	Cardiac/blood	–	1.8 ml
Adrenaline 1:100 000 0.15 mcg/kg	Inotrope	2.7 mcg	0.27 ml
Adrenaline 1:1000 10 mcg/kg	Anaphylaxis	180 mcg IM	0.18 ml
Adrenaline 1:100 000 1 mcg/kg	Anaphylaxis	18 mcg IV	1.8 ml (1:100 000)
Atropine 20 mcg/kg (600 mcg/ml)	HR 60	360 mcg	0.6 ml
Adenosine 150 mcg/kg (3 mg/ml)	SVT	2.7 mg	0.9 ml

OTHER

Cefotaxime 50 mg/kg (100 mg/ml)	Sepsis	900 mg	9 ml
Diazepam IV 0.4 mg/kg (10 mg/ml)	Seizure	7.2 mg (max. 2 doses)	0.72 ml (max. 2 doses)
Nasal fentanyl 1.5 mcg/kg (50 mcg/ml)	Analgesia	27 mcg	0.54 ml
TXA 15 mg/kg (100 mg/ml)	Trauma	270 mg	2.7 ml

5 years – 18 kg

---

5 years – 18 kg

NORMAL VITAL SIGNS

RR	Tidal vol.	HR	Sys. BP
20–30	108 ml	80–135	>90 mmHg

FLUID BOLUS

5 ml/kg	20 ml/kg	Blood – 5 ml/kg bolus
90 ml	360 ml	90 ml

AIRWAY

ETT size	ETT length	Laryngoscopy	Bougie = 10 Ch (paed.) i-gel = 2 (grey)
5.5 cuffed	14.5 cm	Mac 2	

PRE-HOSPITAL EMERGENCY ANAESTHESIA

Fentanyl 3 mcg/kg 50 mcg/ml	54 mcg	1.08 ml
Ketamine 2 mg/kg 10 mg/ml	36 mg	3.6 ml
Rocuronium 1 mg/kg 10 mg/ml	18 mg	1.8 ml

SEDATION

Morphine 0.1 mg/kg 1 mg/ml	1.8 mg	1.8 ml
Midazolam 0.1 mg/kg 1 mg/ml	1.8 mg	1.8 ml
Ketamine 0.5 mg/kg 10 mg/ml	9 mg	0.9 ml

5 years – 18 kg

6 years – 21 kg

NORMAL VITAL SIGNS

RR	Tidal vol.	HR	Sys. BP
20–30	150 ml	80–130	>90 mmHg

FLUID BOLUS

5 ml/kg	105 ml	
20 ml/kg	420 ml	
Blood – 5 ml/kg bolus	105 ml	

AIRWAY

ETT size	5.5 cuffed	
ETT length	15 cm	
Laryngoscopy	Mac 2 or 3	
	Bougie = 10 Ch (paed.)	
	i-gel = 2 (grey)	

PRE-HOSPITAL EMERGENCY ANAESTHESIA

Drug	Dose (conc.)	Amount	Volume
Fentanyl	3 mcg/kg (50 mcg/ml)	63 mcg	1.26 ml
Ketamine	2 mg/kg (10 mg/ml)	42 mg	4.2 ml
Rocuronium	1 mg/kg (10 mg/ml)	21 mg	2.1 ml

SEDATION

Drug	Dose (conc.)	Amount	Volume
Morphine	0.1 mg/kg (1 mg/ml)	2.1 mg	2.1 ml
Midazolam	0.1 mg/kg (1 mg/ml)	2.1 mg	2.1 ml
Ketamine	0.5 mg/kg (10 mg/ml)	10.5 mg	1.05 ml

6 years – 21 kg

FLUID – OTHER

Glucose 10%		2 ml/kg	42 ml
Hypertonic saline		3 ml/kg	63 ml

CARDIOVASCULAR

Drug	Indication	Amount	Volume
Defibrillation 4 J/kg		85 J	
Adrenaline 1:10 000 10 mcg/kg	Arrest	210 mcg	2.1 ml
Amiodarone 5 mg/kg (30 mg/ml)	Arrest	105 mg	3.5 ml
Sodium bicarb. (8.4%)	Arrest/cardiac	21 mmol	21 ml
Calcium chloride (10%)	Cardiac/blood	–	2.1 ml
Adrenaline 1:100 000 0.15 mcg/kg	Inotrope	3.15 mcg	0.32 ml
Adrenaline 1:1000 10 mcg/kg	Anaphylaxis	210 mcg IM	0.21 ml
Adrenaline 1:100 000 1 mcg/kg	Anaphylaxis	21 mcg IV	2.1 ml (1:100 000)
Atropine 20 mcg/kg (600 mcg/ml)	HR 60	420 mcg	0.7 ml
Adenosine 150 mcg/kg (3 mg/ml)	SVT	3.15 mg	1.05 ml

OTHER

Drug	Indication	Amount	Volume
Cefotaxime 50 mg/kg (100 mg/ml)	Sepsis	1050 mg	10.5 ml
Diazepam IV 0.4 mg/kg (10 mg/ml)	Seizure	8.4 mg (max. 2 doses)	0.84 ml (max. 2 doses)
Nasal fentanyl 1.5 mcg/kg (50 mcg/ml)	Analgesia	31.5 mcg	0.63 ml
TXA 15 mg/kg (100 mg/ml)	Trauma	315 mg	3.15 ml

6 years – 21 kg

7 years – 23 kg

NORMAL VITAL SIGNS

RR	Tidal vol.	HR	Sys. BP
20–30	138 ml	80–130	>90 mmHg

FLUID BOLUS

5 ml/kg	10 ml/kg	20 ml/kg	Blood – 5 ml/kg bolus
115 ml	230 ml	460 ml	115 ml

AIRWAY

ETT size	ETT length	Laryngoscopy
6 cuffed	15.5 cm	Mac 2 or 3
	Bougie = 15 Ch (adult)	
	i-gel = 2 (grey)	

PRE-HOSPITAL EMERGENCY ANAESTHESIA

Fentanyl	3 mcg/kg / 50 mcg/ml	69 mcg	1.38 ml
Ketamine	2 mg/kg / 10 mg/ml	46 mg	4.6 ml
Rocuronium	1 mg/kg / 10 mg/ml	23 mg	2.3 ml

SEDATION

Morphine	0.1 mg/kg / 1 mg/ml	2.3 mg	2.3 ml
Midazolam	0.1 mg/kg / 1 mg/ml	2.3 mg	2.3 ml
Ketamine	0.5 mg/kg / 10 mg/ml	11.5 mg	1.15 ml

7 years – 23 kg

FLUID – OTHER

Glucose 10%	2 ml/kg	46 ml
Hypertonic saline	3 ml/kg	69 ml

CARDIOVASCULAR

Defibrillation 4 J/kg	Arrest		90 J
Adrenaline 1:10 000 10 mcg/kg	Arrest	230 mcg	2.3 ml
Amiodarone 5 mg/kg (30 mg/ml)	Arrest	115 mg	3.83 ml
Sodium bicarb. (8.4%)	Arrest/cardiac	23 mmol	23 ml
Calcium chloride (10%)	Cardiac/blood	–	2.3 ml
Adrenaline 1:100 000 0.15 mcg/kg	Inotrope	3.45 mcg	0.35 ml
Adrenaline 1:1000 10 mcg/kg	Anaphylaxis	230 mcg IM	0.23 ml
Adrenaline 1:100 000 1 mcg/kg	Anaphylaxis	23 mcg IV	2.3 ml (1:100 000)
Atropine 20 mcg/kg (600 mcg/ml)	HR 60	460 mcg	0.77 ml
Adenosine 150 mcg/kg (3 mg/ml)	SVT	3.45 mg	1.15 ml

OTHER

Cefotaxime 50 mg/kg (100 mg/ml)	Sepsis	1150 mg	11.5 ml
Diazepam IV 0.4 mg/kg (10 mg/ml)	Seizure	9.2 mg (max. 2 doses)	0.92 ml (max. 2 doses)
Nasal fentanyl 1.5 mcg/kg (50 mcg/ml)	Analgesia	34.5 mcg	0.69 ml
TXA 15 mg/kg (100 mg/ml)	Trauma	345 mg	3.45 ml

7 years – 23 kg

8 years – 25 kg

FLUID – OTHER

Glucose 10%	2 ml/kg	50 ml
Hypertonic saline	3 ml/kg	75 ml

CARDIOVASCULAR

Defibrillation 4 J/kg		100 J	
Adrenaline 1:10 000 10 mcg/kg	Arrest	250 mcg	2.5 ml
Amiodarone 5 mg/kg (30 mg/ml)	Arrest	125 mg	4.17 ml
Sodium bicarb. (8.4%)	Arrest/cardiac	25 mmol	25 ml
Calcium chloride (10%)	Cardiac/blood	–	2.5 ml
Adrenaline 1:100 000 0.15 mcg/kg	Inotrope	3.75 mcg	0.38 ml
Adrenaline 1:1000 10 mcg/kg	Anaphylaxis	250 mcg IM	0.25 ml
Adrenaline 1:100 000 1 mcg/kg	Anaphylaxis	25 mcg IV	2.5 ml (1:100 000)
Atropine 20 mcg/kg (600 mcg/ml)	HR 60	600 mcg	1 ml
Adenosine 150 mcg/kg (3 mg/ml)	SVT	3.75 mg	1.25 ml

OTHER

Cefotaxime 50 mg/kg (100 mg/ml)	Sepsis	1250 mg	12.5 ml
Diazepam IV 0.4 mg/kg (10 mg/ml)	Seizure	10 mg (max. 2 doses)	1 ml (max. 2 doses)
Nasal fentanyl 1.5 mcg/kg (50 mcg/ml)	Analgesia	37.5 mcg	0.75 ml
TXA 15 mg/kg (100 mg/ml)	Trauma	375 mg	3.75 ml

8 years – 25 kg

---

8 years – 25 kg

NORMAL VITAL SIGNS

RR	Tidal vol.	HR	Sys. BP
15–25	150 ml	70–120	>90 mmHg

FLUID BOLUS

5 ml/kg	10 ml/kg	20 ml/kg	Blood – 5 ml/kg bolus
125 ml	250 ml	500 ml	125 ml

AIRWAY

ETT size	ETT length	Laryngoscopy	
6 cuffed	16 cm	Mac 3	Bougie = 15 Ch (adult); i-gel = 2.5 (white)

PRE-HOSPITAL EMERGENCY ANAESTHESIA

Fentanyl	3 mcg/kg 50 mcg/ml	75 mcg	1.5 ml
Ketamine	2 mg/kg 10 mg/ml	50 mg	5 ml
Rocuronium	1 mg/kg 10 mg/ml	25 mg	2.5 ml

SEDATION

Morphine	0.1 mg/kg 1 mg/ml	2.5 mg	2.5 ml
Midazolam	0.1 mg/kg 1 mg/ml	2.5 mg	2.5 ml
Ketamine	0.5 mg/kg 10 mg/ml	12.5 mg	1.25 ml

8 years – 25 kg

9 years – 28 kg

NORMAL VITAL SIGNS

RR	Tidal vol.	HR	Sys. BP
15–25	168 ml	70–120	>90 mmHg

FLUID BOLUS

5 ml/kg	10 ml/kg	20 ml/kg	Blood – 5 ml/kg bolus
140 ml	280 ml	560 ml	140 ml

AIRWAY

ETT size	ETT length	Laryngoscopy	Mac 3
6.5 cuffed	16.5 cm	Bougie = 15 Ch (adult)	i-gel = 2.5 (white)

PRE-HOSPITAL EMERGENCY ANAESTHESIA

Drug	Dose / conc.		
Fentanyl	3 mcg/kg / 50 mcg/ml	84 mcg	1.68 ml
Ketamine	2 mg/kg / 10 mg/ml	56 mg	5.6 ml
Rocuronium	1 mg/kg / 10 mg/ml	28 mg	2.8 ml

SEDATION

Morphine	0.1 mg/kg / 1 mg/ml	2.8 mg	2.8 ml
Midazolam	0.1 mg/kg / 1 mg/ml	2.8 mg	2.8 ml
Ketamine	0.5 mg/kg / 10 mg/ml	14 mg	1.4 ml

9 years – 28 kg

FLUID – OTHER

Glucose 10%	2 ml/kg	56 ml
Hypertonic saline	3 ml/kg	84 ml

CARDIOVASCULAR

Drug	Indication	Dose	Volume
Defibrillation 4 J/kg	Arrest	110 J	
Adrenaline 1:10 000 10 mcg/kg	Arrest	280 mcg	2.8 ml
Amiodarone 5 mg/kg (30 mg/ml)	Arrest	140 mg	4.67 ml
Sodium bicarb. (8.4%)	Arrest/cardiac	28 mmol	28 ml
Calcium chloride (10%)	Cardiac/blood	–	2.8 ml
Adrenaline 1:100 000 0.15 mcg/kg	Inotrope	4.2 mcg	0.42 ml
Adrenaline 1:1000 10 mcg/kg	Anaphylaxis	280 mcg IM	0.28 ml
Adrenaline 1:100 000 1 mcg/kg	Anaphylaxis	28 mcg IV	2.8 ml (1:100 000)
Atropine 20 mcg/kg (600 mcg/ml)	HR 60	600 mcg	1 ml
Adenosine 150 mcg/kg (3 mg/ml)	SVT	4.2 mg	1.4 ml

OTHER

Cefotaxime 50 mg/kg (100 mg/ml)	Sepsis	1400 mg	14 ml
Diazepam IV 0.4 mg/kg (10 mg/ml)	Seizure	10 mg (max. 2 doses)	1 ml (max. 2 doses)
Nasal fentanyl 1.5 mcg/kg (50 mcg/ml)	Analgesia	42 mcg	0.84 ml
TXA 15 mg/kg (100 mg/ml)	Trauma	420 mg	4.2 ml

9 years – 28 kg

10 years – 31 kg

NORMAL VITAL SIGNS

RR	Tidal vol.	HR	Sys. BP
15–25	186 ml	70–120	>90 mmHg

FLUID BOLUS

Blood – 5 ml/kg bolus	155 ml	
20 ml/kg	620 ml	
5 ml/kg	155 ml	

AIRWAY

	ETT length	Laryngoscopy	Mac 3
ETT size	17 cm	Bougie = 15 Ch (adult)	
6.5 cuffed		i-gel = 2.5 (white)	

PRE-HOSPITAL EMERGENCY ANAESTHESIA

Fentanyl	3 mcg/kg	93 mcg	1.86 ml
	50 mcg/ml		
Ketamine	2 mg/kg	62 mg	6.2 ml
	10 mg/ml		
Rocuronium	1 mg/kg	31 mg	3.1 ml
	10 mg/ml		

SEDATION

Morphine	0.1 mg/kg	3.1 mg	3.1 ml
	1 mg/ml		
Midazolam	0.1 mg/kg	3.1 mg	3.1 ml
	1 mg/ml		
Ketamine	0.5 mg/kg	15.5 mg	1.55 ml
	10 mg/ml		

10 years   31 kg

---

10 years – 31 kg

FLUID – OTHER

Glucose 10%	2 ml/kg	62 ml
Hypertonic saline	3 ml/kg	93 ml

CARDIOVASCULAR

Defibrillation 4 J/kg	Arrest		125 J
Adrenaline 1:10 000 10 mcg/kg	Arrest	310 mcg	3.1 ml
Amiodarone 5 mg/kg (30 mg/ml)	Arrest	155 mg	5.17 ml
Sodium bicarb. (8.4%)	Arrest/cardiac	31 mmol	31 ml
Calcium chloride (10%)	Cardiac/blood	–	3.1 ml
Adrenaline 1:100 000 0.15 mcg/kg	Inotrope	4.65 mcg	0.46 ml
Adrenaline 1:1000 10 mcg/kg	Anaphylaxis	310 mcg IM	0.31 ml
Adrenaline 1:100 000 1 mcg/kg	Anaphylaxis	31 mcg IV	3.1 ml (1:100 000)
Atropine 20 mcg/kg (600 mcg/ml)	HR 60	600 mcg	1 ml
Adenosine 150 mcg/kg (3 mg/ml)	SVT	4.65 mg	1.55 ml

OTHER

Cefotaxime 50 mg/kg (100 mg/ml)	Sepsis	1550 mg	15.5 ml
Diazepam IV 0.4 mg/kg (10 mg/ml)	Seizure	10 mg (max. 2 doses)	1 ml (max. 2 doses)
Nasal fentanyl 1.5 mcg/kg (50 mcg/ml)	Analgesia	46.5 mcg	0.93 ml
TXA 15 mg/kg (100 mg/ml)	Trauma	465 mg	4.65 ml

10 years – 31 kg

11 years – 35 kg

NORMAL VITAL SIGNS

RR	Tidal vol.	HR	Sys. BP
15–25	210 ml	70–120	>90 mmHg

FLUID BOLUS

5 ml/kg	10 ml/kg	20 ml/kg	Blood – 5 ml/kg bolus
175 ml	350 ml	700 ml	175 ml

AIRWAY

ETT size	ETT length	Laryngoscopy
7 cuffed	17.5 cm	Mac 3
	Bougie = 15 Ch (adult)	i-gel = 3 (yellow)

PRE-HOSPITAL EMERGENCY ANAESTHESIA

Fentanyl	3 mcg/kg	105 mcg	2.1 ml
	50 mcg/ml		
Ketamine	2 mg/kg	70 mg	7 ml
	10 mg/ml		
Rocuronium	1 mg/kg	35 mg	3.5 ml
	10 mg/ml		

SEDATION

Morphine	0.1 mg/kg	3.5 mg	3.5 ml
	1 mg/ml		
Midazolam	0.1 mg/kg	3.5 mg	3.5 ml
	1 mg/ml		
Ketamine	0.5 mg/kg	17.5 mg	1.75 ml
	10 mg/ml		

11 years – 35 kg

---

11 years – 35 kg

FLUID – OTHER

Glucose 10%	2 ml/kg	70 ml
Hypertonic saline	3 ml/kg	105 ml

CARDIOVASCULAR

Defibrillation 4 J/kg	Arrest	140 J	
Adrenaline 1:10 000 10 mcg/kg	Arrest	350 mcg	3.5 ml
Amiodarone 5 mg/kg (30 mg/ml)	Arrest	175 mg	5.83 ml
Sodium bicarb. (8.4%)	Arrest/cardiac	35 mmol	35 ml
Calcium chloride (10%)	Cardiac/blood	–	3.5 ml
Adrenaline 1:100 000 0.15 mcg/kg	Inotrope	5.25 mcg	0.53 ml
Adrenaline 1:1000 10 mcg/kg	Anaphylaxis	350 mcg IM	0.35 ml
Adrenaline 1:100 000 1 mcg/kg	Anaphylaxis	35 mcg IV	3.5 ml (1:100 000)
Atropine 20 mcg/kg (600 mcg/ml)	HR 60	600 mcg	1 ml
Adenosine 150 mcg/kg (3 mg/ml)	SVT	5.25 mg	1.75 ml

OTHER

Cefotaxime 50 mg/kg (100 mg/ml)	Sepsis	1750 mg	17.5 ml
Diazepam IV 0.4 mg/kg (10 mg/ml)	Seizure	10 mg (max. 2 doses)	1 ml (max. 2 doses)
Nasal fentanyl 1.5 mcg/kg (50 mcg/ml)	Analgesia	52.5 mcg	1.05 ml
TXA 15 mg/kg (100 mg/ml)	Trauma	525 mg	5.25 ml

11 years – 35 kg

12 years – 43 kg

NORMAL VITAL SIGNS

RR	Tidal vol.	HR	Sys. BP
12–24	258 ml	65–115	>100 mmHg

FLUID BOLUS

5 ml/kg	20 ml/kg	Blood – 5 ml/kg bolus
215 ml	860 ml	215 ml

AIRWAY

ETT size	ETT length	Laryngoscopy	Mac 3
7 cuffed	18 cm	Bougie = 15 Ch (adult)	
		i-gel = 3 (yellow)	

PRE-HOSPITAL EMERGENCY ANAESTHESIA

Fentanyl	3 mcg/kg 50 mcg/ml	129 mcg	2.58 ml
Ketamine	2 mg/kg 10 mg/ml	86 mg	8.6 ml
Rocuronium	1 mg/kg 10 mg/ml	43 mg	4.3 ml

SEDATION

Morphine	0.1 mg/kg 1 mg/ml	4.3 mg	4.3 ml
Midazolam	0.1 mg/kg 1 mg/ml	4.3 mg	4.3 ml
Ketamine	0.5 mg/kg 10 mg/ml	21.5 mg	2.15 ml

12 years – 43 kg

FLUID – OTHER

Glucose 10%	2 ml/kg	86 ml
Hypertonic saline	3 ml/kg	129 ml

CARDIOVASCULAR

Defibrillation 4 J/kg	Arrest	170 J	
Adrenaline 1:10 000 10 mcg/kg	Arrest	430 mcg	4.3 ml
Amiodarone 5 mg/kg (30 mg/ml)	Arrest	215 mg	7.17 ml
Sodium bicarb. (8.4%)	Arrest/cardiac	43 mmol	43 ml
Calcium chloride (10%)	Cardiac/blood	–	4.3 ml
Adrenaline 1:100 000 0.15 mcg/kg	Inotrope	6.45 mcg	0.65 ml
Adrenaline 1:1000 10 mcg/kg	Anaphylaxis	430 mcg IM	0.43 ml
Adrenaline 1:100 000 1 mcg/kg	Anaphylaxis	43 mcg IV	4.3 ml (1:100 000)
Atropine 20 mcg/kg (600 mcg/ml)	HR 60	600 mcg	1 ml
Adenosine 150 mcg/kg (3 mg/ml)	SVT	6.45 mg	2.15 ml

OTHER

Cefotaxime 50 mg/kg (100 mg/ml)	Sepsis	2150 mg	21.5 ml
Diazepam IV 0.4 mg/kg (10 mg/ml)	Seizure	10 mg (max. 2 doses)	1 ml (max. 2 doses)
Nasal fentanyl 1.5 mcg/kg (50 mcg/ml)	Analgesia	64.5 mcg	1.29 ml
TXA 15 mg/kg (100 mg/ml)	Trauma	645 mg	6.45 ml

12 years – 43 kg

14 years – 50 kg

FLUID – OTHER

Glucose 10%	2 ml/kg	100 ml
Hypertonic saline	3 ml/kg	150 ml

CARDIOVASCULAR

Defibrillation 4 J/kg		200 J	
Adrenaline 1:10 000 10 mcg/kg	Arrest	500 mcg	5 ml
Amiodarone 5 mg/kg (30 mg/ml)	Arrest	250 mg	8.33 ml
Sodium bicarb. (8.4%)	Arrest/cardiac	50 mmol	50 ml
Calcium chloride (10%)	Cardiac/blood	–	5 ml
Adrenaline 1:100 000 0.15 mcg/kg	Inotrope	7.5 mcg	0.75 ml
Adrenaline 1:1000 10 mcg/kg	Anaphylaxis	500 mcg IM	0.5 ml
Adrenaline 1:100 000 1 mcg/kg	Anaphylaxis	50 mcg IV	5 ml (1:100 000)
Atropine 20 mcg/kg (600 mcg/ml)	HR 60	600 mcg	1 ml
Adenosine 150 mcg/kg (3 mg/ml)	SVT	7.5 mg	2.5 ml

OTHER

Cefotaxime 50 mg/kg (100 mg/ml)	Sepsis	2500 mg	25 ml
Diazepam IV 0.4 mg/kg (10 mg/ml)	Seizure	10 mg (max. 2 doses)	1 ml (max. 2 doses)
Nasal fentanyl 1.5 mcg/kg (50 mcg/ml)	Analgesia	75 mcg	1.5 ml
TXA 15 mg/kg (100 mg/ml)	Trauma	750 mg	7.5 ml

14 years – 50 kg

---

14 years – 50 kg

NORMAL VITAL SIGNS

RR	Tidal vol.	HR	Sys. BP
12–24	300 ml	65–115	>100 mmHg

FLUID BOLUS

5 ml/kg	10 ml/kg	20 ml/kg	Blood – 5 ml/kg bolus
250 ml	500 ml	1000 ml	250 ml

AIRWAY

ETT size	ETT length	Laryngoscopy	Mac 3
7 cuffed	19 cm	Bougie = 15 Ch (adult)	
		i-gel = 3 (yellow)	

PRE-HOSPITAL EMERGENCY ANAESTHESIA

Fentanyl	3 mcg/kg / 50 mcg/ml	150 mcg	3 ml
Ketamine	2 mg/kg / 10 mg/ml	100 mg	10 ml
Rocuronium	1 mg/kg / 10 mg/ml	50 mg	5 ml

SEDATION

Morphine	0.1 mg/kg / 1 mg/ml	5 mg	5 ml
Midazolam	0.1 mg/kg / 1 mg/ml	5 mg	5 ml
Ketamine	0.5 mg/kg / 10 mg/ml	25 mg	2.5 ml

14 years – 50 kg

Critical Care Formulary			
Drug	**Concentration**	**Dose**	**Volume**
ALTERNATE INDUCTION AGENTS			
Propofol	10 mg/ml	**2 mg/kg**	**0.2 ml/kg**
VASOPRESSORS			
Metaraminol	0.5 mg/ml	**0.01 mg/kg**	**0.02 ml/kg**
ASTHMA			
Hydrocortisone	100 mg/ml	**4 mg/kg**	**0.04 ml/kg**
Salbutamol BOLUS (over 15 min)	10 mg in 50 ml 0.9% saline	**15 mcg/kg (only in age 2+ years)**	**0.075 ml/kg**
Magnesium sulphate	200 mg/ml	**40 mg/kg (over 20 min)**	**0.75 ml/kg**
Magnesium sulphate	200 mg/ml	**150 mg NEBULISED**	**0.75 ml added to nebuliser**
Consider ketamine 0.1–2 mg/kg boluses titrated to effect in extremis			
LOCAL ANAESTHESIA			
Bupivacaine	5 mg/ml	**Max. 2 mg/kg**	**0.4 ml/kg**
Lignocaine	10 mg/ml	**Max. 3 mg/kg**	**0.3 ml/kg**
ANALGESIA			
Morphine	10 mg/ml	**0.1–0.2 mg/kg**	**1 mg/ml = 0.1 ml/kg**
Ketamine	10 mg/ml	**0.1–0.3 mg/kg**	**0.01–0.03 ml/kg**
Paracetamol	10 mg/ml	**15 mg/kg**	**1.5 ml/kg**
REVERSAL OF OPIOID/BENZODIAZEPINE			
Naloxone	400 mcg/ml	**100 mcg/kg**	**0.25 ml/kg**
Flumazenil	100 mcg/ml	**10–50 mcg/kg**	**0.1 ml/kg**
ANTIEMETIC			
Ondansetron	2 mg/ml	**0.1 mg/kg**	**0.05 ml/kg**
Cyclizine	25 mg/ml	**<6 years = 0.5 mg/kg**	**0.02 ml/kg**
Cyclizine	25 mg/ml	**6–12 years = 25 mg >12years = 50 mg**	**0.5 ml 1 ml**
Critical Care Formulary			

Paediatric GCS		
Eye opening		
Spontaneously		4
Response to voice		3
Response to pain		2
None		1
Verbal		
Under 5	Over 5	
Alert, coos or babbles words or sentences to usual ability	Orientated	5
Less than usual ability, irritable cry	Confused	4
Cries to pain	Inappropriate words	3
Moans to pain	Incomprehensible	2
No response to pain		1
Motor		
Under 5	Over 5	
Normal spontaneous movements	Obeys commands	6
Under 9/12	Over 9/12	
Withdraws to touch	Localises to pain	5
Withdraws from nailbed pain		4
Flexion to supraorbital pain (decorticate)		3
Extension to supraorbital pain (decrerebrate)		2
No response to supraorbital pain (flaccid)		1
Paediatric GCS		

Sources: JRCALC Clinical Practice Guidelines 2016, Advanced Paediatric Life Support Manual 6e & cBNF

Developed by Dr Jim Blackburn / Dr James Tooley
from designs by Karel Habig & Dr Chris Hill

Kindly supported & printed by:

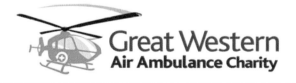

Great Western
Air Ambulance Charity

Index